Contents

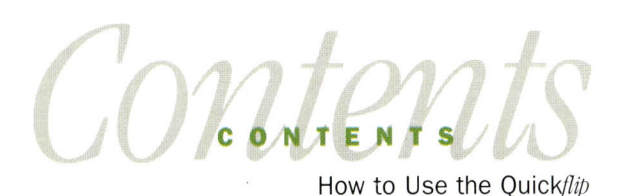

How to Use the Quick*flip*	2
The Quick*flip* Flavors	3
The Pantry	4
Pasta *Tips & Recipes*	5-6
Pizza *Tips & Recipes*	7-8
Sauté *Tips & Recipes*	9-10
Stir Fry *Tips & Recipes*	11-12
Oven Baked *Tips & Recipes*	13-14
Soup *Tips & Recipes*	15-16
Grains *Tips & Recipes*	17-18
Veggies *Tips & Recipes*	19-20
Chicken/Fish/Soy *Tips & Recipes*	21-22
Dessert *Tips & Recipes*	23-24
Guide to Ingredients	25
Nutritional Analyses	26-29
Food & Nutrition Resources	30

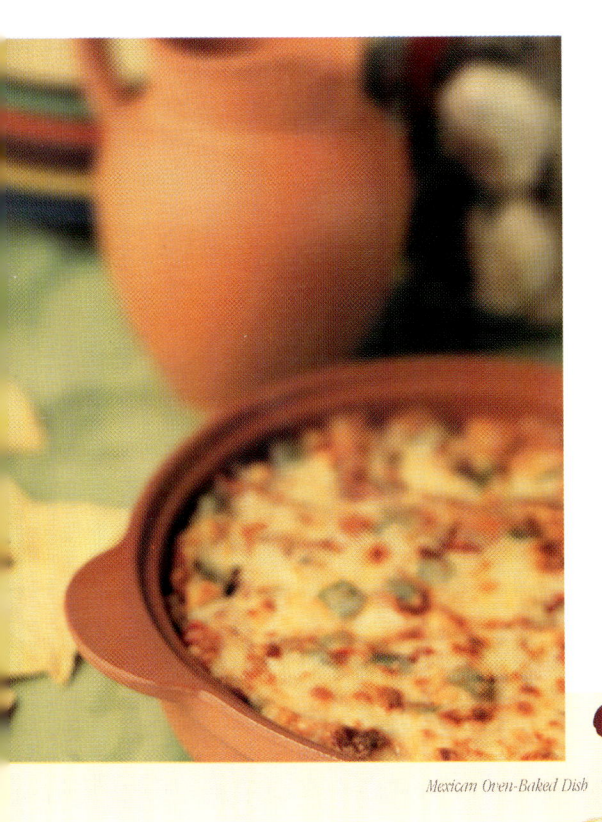

Mexican Oven-Baked Dish

"I want to eat healthier meals, but I need new ideas for what to make."

After hearing comments like these over and over from people I counsel in my nutrition practice, I realized that we need more than nutrition facts to improve our eating habits. We need tools that will help us bridge the gap between what we know we should be eating and what we actually eat. As a Registered Dietitian with training at the Culinary

"I want to prepare healthier meals, but I don't have the time."

Institute of America, I wanted to make it easy and convenient for people to prepare nutritious, good-tasting meals.

The **Quick***flip*™ to *Delicious Dinners* does this by removing the clutter and confusion of countless recipes and organizing them into a simple, logical system. I hope you'll enjoy and benefit from the **Quick***flip*.

Eileen

How to Use the Quick*flip*™

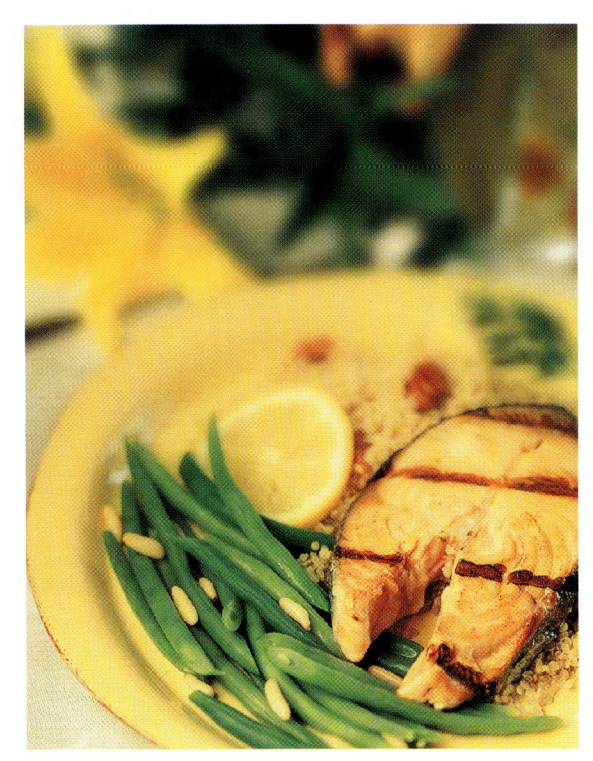

French salmon, Southwestern Quinoa

Discover an innovative system that lets you turn a basic recipe into 5 delicious variations – simply by changing a few ingredients.

The **Quick***flip* to Delicious Dinners was designed to simplify meal preparation. First stock your *Pantry* with the items listed on page 4. Next, select a recipe and decide which variation you would like to prepare. Now, all you need to prepare that recipe are the fresh ingredients. These are shown in green – that's your *Shopping List* for that meal.

Each recipe has *Cooking Directions* at the top of the page. This one set of instructions is used to make each of the *International Variations* of that recipe. On the page before the recipe, you will find some *Tips and Hints* for preparing the recipes in that group.

There is an additional *Guide to Ingredients* on page 25, as well as *Nutrition Facts* and *Food Exchange* information on pages 26-29. Feel free to adjust the recipes to your own personal taste. This is a system that encourages you to be creative.

It's as simple as that. You're on your way to good eating.

The Quick*flip* *Flavors*
healthy ingredients from around the world

When you think of a healthy diet, do you think of bland, tasteless food and a long list of all the delicious foods you shouldn't eat? Fortunately, with our better understanding of nutrition today, you no longer have to think that way. Today's nutritional guidelines are not based on narrow food choices and "dieting," but on enjoying a wide variety of delicious healthy foods in moderation.

The "new" nutritional guidelines are actually not new at all. They are based on traditional diets from around the world that we now know are linked with good health. The world's cuisines are rich in flavors and healthy ingredients. Adding these healthy foods may be just as important, if not more so, than limiting the foods we shouldn't eat.

The **Quick***flip* uses a wide variety of wholesome ingredients from this global pantry. Recipes emphasize plant foods, including grains, fruits, vegetables, beans, nuts, and herbs and spices. In addition to containing vitamins, minerals, and fiber, these foods are rich sources of health-promoting phytochemicals. They also offer a wonderful array of flavors, colors and textures.

The Quick*flip* recipes incorporate the best of diets from around the world and use common, easy to find ingredients that are combined in creative ways. Many of the recipes use vegetables generously – even as a flavoring for rice dishes. Fruits and nuts are used to make appetizing desserts.

The Quick*flip* recipes include protein sources such as chicken and fish in the smaller amounts recommended for good health or they are optional. The recipes give you the flexibility to make vegetarian dishes or to increase, decrease, add or delete ingredients to your personal taste.

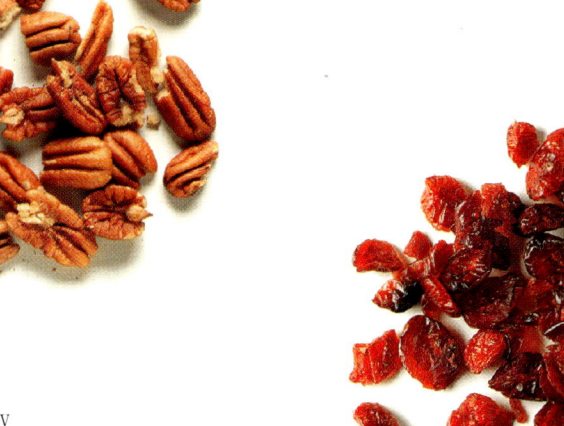

Since the type of fat we eat may be more important for good health than how much fat we eat, the Quick*flip* recipes use healthy sources of fat such as olive oil and nuts in moderate amounts.

As you flip through the Quick*flip's* recipe pages you'll quickly see that a healthy diet is not one that restricts and limits foods. Instead, it's one that expands the choices and adds variety, nutrients and flavor.

Perhaps the best thing about using the Quick*flip* is that it makes it easy to prepare healthy meals. You'll have more time to relax and enjoy what you eat – another important part of a healthy lifestyle!

THE PANTRY

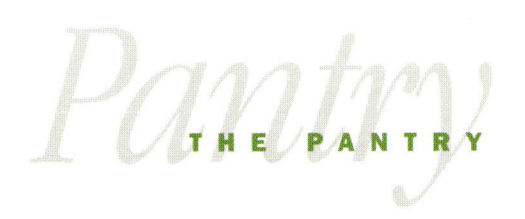

A thoughtfully stocked pantry is the backbone of the kitchen.

This pantry list was devised for these recipes, but you'll find it helpful for making many other meals. Pantry items are listed in purple in each recipe. Ingredients that are best purchased fresh are listed in green.

Feel free to substitute items that you have on hand and increase or decrease the measure of ingredients to suit your own tastes. The **Quick***flip*™ system invites you to try new combinations.

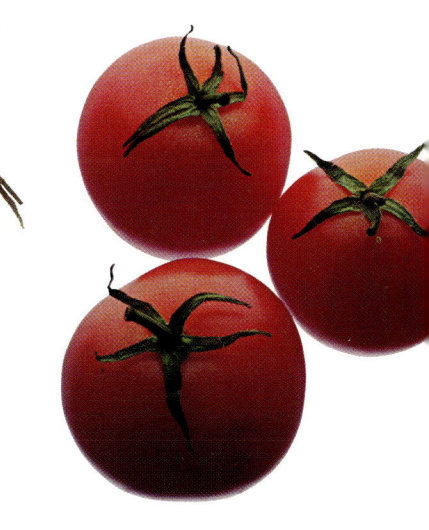

Canned Goods
Apple juice concentrate
Artichoke hearts
Beans - black, garbanzo, pinto, refried, cannellini (or dried beans)
Broth - vegetable or chicken (or home made)
Evaporated skim milk
Green chilies
Mandarin oranges
Pineapple tidbits
Tomatoes
Tomato juice
Tomato paste
Tomato puree
Tomato sauce
Water chestnuts

Dried/Frozen Fruits and Vegetables
Raisins
Sun-dried tomatoes
Frozen blackberries, blueberries, strawberries

Grains/Starches
Beans - see canned goods
Lentils
Polenta (corn grits)
Couscous
Flour – if making your own pizza crust
Pasta – several varieties perhaps including: bow tie, fettuccine, lasagna, penne, shells, udon noodles, ziti
Quinoa
Rice – brown, white, basmati, jasmine

Nuts and Seeds
(These can be stored in airtight containers in the refrigerator or freezer)
Almonds
Peanuts
Pine nuts
Walnuts
Sesame seeds
Peanut butter
Tahini (ground sesame seeds)

Oils
Olive, dark sesame, canola

Vinegars
Balsamic, red wine, rice

Wines
Red and white

Spices, Flavorings, and Condiments
(The following items are used in the recipes, but you can edit this list to your liking.)

Allspice, almond flavor, basil, cayenne pepper, cardamom, chili powder, cinnamon, cloves, coriander, cumin, curry, dill, garlic cloves, garlic powder, marjoram, nutmeg, oregano, pepper, red pepper flakes, salt, tarragon, thyme, turmeric

Cornstarch, honey, prepared mustard, mirin, olives, salsa, soy sauce or tamari, Thai chili paste, Thai fish sauce, Worcestershire sauce

Pasta

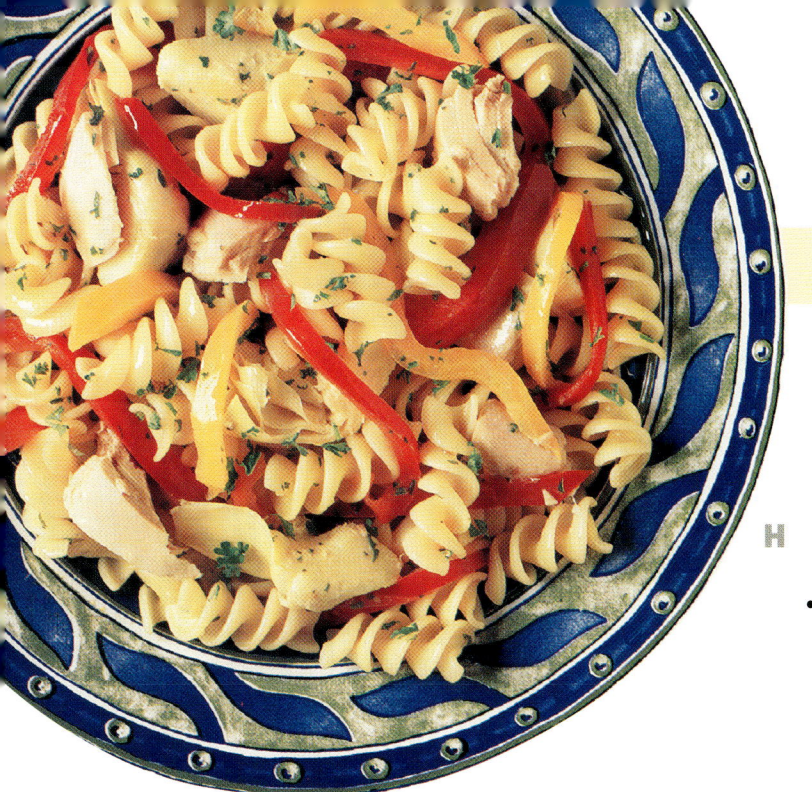

Spanish Pasta

Tasty
HINTS

- For variety and added nutrients, try whole grain pastas, flavored pastas, and pastas made from other flours such as corn, rice, quinoa, and amaranth.

- Asian noodles made from buckwheat, rice, wheat, or beans offer additional flavor and texture options. Udon noodles are made from whole wheat flour.

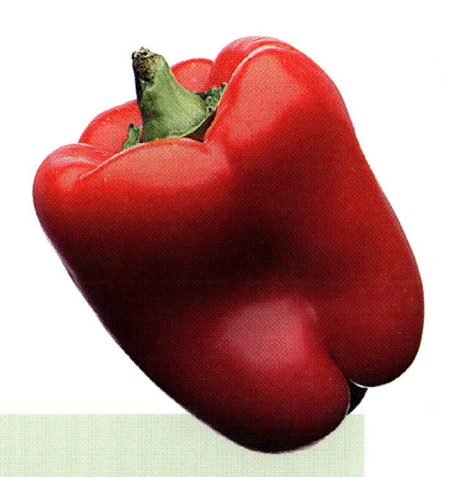

Healthy
HINTS

- Grains and grain products such as pasta should be the major source of calories in our diet. Six to eleven servings each day is recommended with at least three being whole grains. A serving is equivalent to one slice of bread or 1/2 cup of cereal, pasta, rice or other grain. Most grains have less than 200 calories per cooked cup, no cholesterol, only a trace of fat, and contain many nutrients.

- Most fresh pastas are made with eggs and contain 55 mg of cholesterol and slightly more fat per cooked cup than dried varieties.

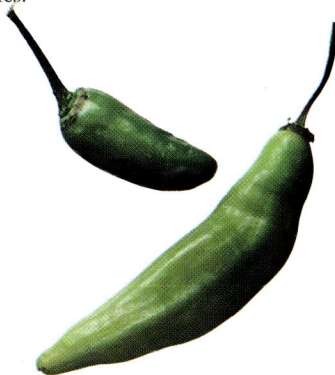

How to Make Lower Fat Sauces

Any of these methods can be used to make flavorful sauces:

Substitute evaporated skim milk for cream.

Add 1/3 cup nonfat dry milk to one cup of skim milk. Use in place of cream or whole milk.

For creamy chicken, fish, or beef flavored sauces, add 1/3 cup nonfat dry milk to broth and add a little wine or sherry.

Cornstarch or flour can be used as thickeners instead of higher fat ingredients. Flour can be used to thicken gravies and white or brown sauces, while cornstarch works well for translucent sauces. To thicken 1 1/2 - 2 cups of liquid, mix 1 T. cornstarch or 2-4 T. flour with a small amount of cold liquid and add to the sauce. When cornstarch is used, add the mixture to the sauce during the last 2 minutes of cooking. When using flour, allow the sauce to simmer at least 3 minutes after adding the flour mixture.

Extra seasonings can be used to add flavor to low-fat sauces.

Five International Variations

Pasta

4 to 6 Servings

Cooking Directions for the Basic Recipe

1. Cook pasta according to package directions.
2. Prepare all vegetables and seasonings.
3. Place cooking liquid in saucepan over medium-high heat.
4. Add vegetables and seasonings and cook for 3-7 minutes.
5. Add the ad lib and cook for 3-5 minutes or until all food is heated and cooked to desired tenderness.
6. Pour vegetable mixture over the hot pasta.

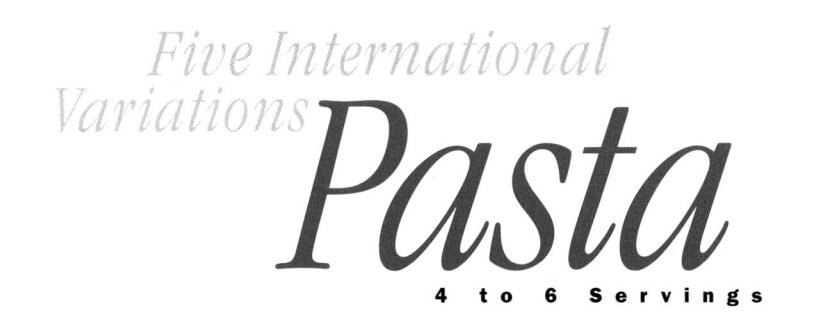

Ingredients	ASIAN	FRENCH	ITALIAN	MEXICAN	SPANISH
Pasta	12 oz. udon noodles (or linguine)[g]	12 oz. of pasta shells[g]	12 oz. ziti[g]	12 oz. of bow tie pasta[g]	12 oz. penne pasta[g]
Vegetables	1 cup each: carrots, thinly sliced scallions, chopped snow peas, bean sprouts, 2 cups mushrooms, sliced	1 cup onions, diced 2 cups each: zucchini, plum tomatoes, mushrooms, chopped	3 cups tomatoes, chopped 2 cups zucchini, sliced 1 cup onions, finely chopped	3 cups tomatoes, diced 1 cup onion, finely diced 7 oz. can green chilies	2 cups red pepper 1 cup yellow or green pepper (all peppers cut in thin strips) 1 cup onion, thinly sliced 1 cup of artichoke hearts, quartered
Seasonings	2 tsp. garlic, minced 1 T. fresh ginger, grated 1/4 tsp. red pepper flakes	1 T. garlic, minced 2 T. fresh basil, chopped 1/4 cup fresh parsley, chopped 1/4 tsp. pepper salt	2 tsp. garlic, minced 2-3 anchovies, optional 1 tsp. oregano 1/2 tsp. sage 1/2 tsp. marjoram	1 T. garlic, chopped 1/4 tsp. cumin salt	2 tsp. garlic, minced 1 tsp. thyme 1/4 cup fresh parsley, chopped 1/4 tsp. pepper salt
Cooking Liquid	1 T. sesame oil 3 T. soy sauce 1/3 cup rice vinegar 1/3 cup white wine or broth	1/2 cup clam juice 1/2 cup white wine	3/4 cup broth 1/2 cup white wine 1 T. olive oil 2 T. tomato paste	1/2 cup broth and 1 cup salsa	1 T. olive oil 3/4 cup broth 2 T. lemon juice
Ad Lib[a]	1 cup cooked chicken, cut into strips or 2 T. peanuts	8 oz. bay scallops or any firm white fish cut into 1 inch chunks (e.g. cod, snapper, grouper) 1 cup evaporated skim milk mixed with 3 T. flour 1/4 cup parmesan cheese, optional	1 cup cooked cannellini beans[g]	1 cup cooked, diced chicken or cooked pinto beans[g]	6 oz. tuna or 1/3 cup parmesan cheese

[g] See guide on page 25.

[a] Use one of the suggested ingredients or substitute your own special ingredient.

6

Pizza

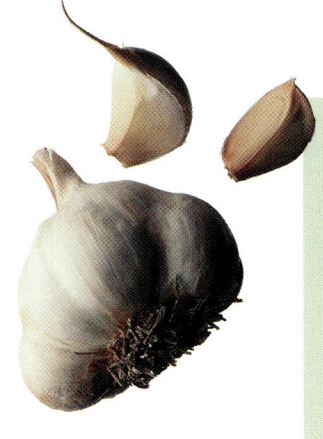

Quick Pizza Crust
2 cups all-purpose flour
1 pkg. Rapid-Rise yeast
1/2 tsp. sugar
3/4 tsp. salt
3/4 cups warm water
1 tsp. olive oil

In food processor, combine the flour, yeast, sugar and salt. Mix the warm water (125 degrees) and oil and gradually add to the food processor while the motor is running.

Process until the dough forms a ball, adding up to 2 T. cold water, if necessary. Process an additional minute to knead. Turn out onto a lightly floured surface. Cover with plastic wrap and let rest for 10 minutes. Shape into one large crust or 4-6 individual crusts.

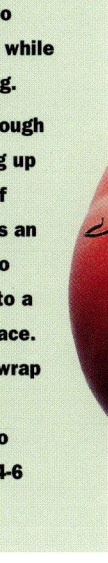

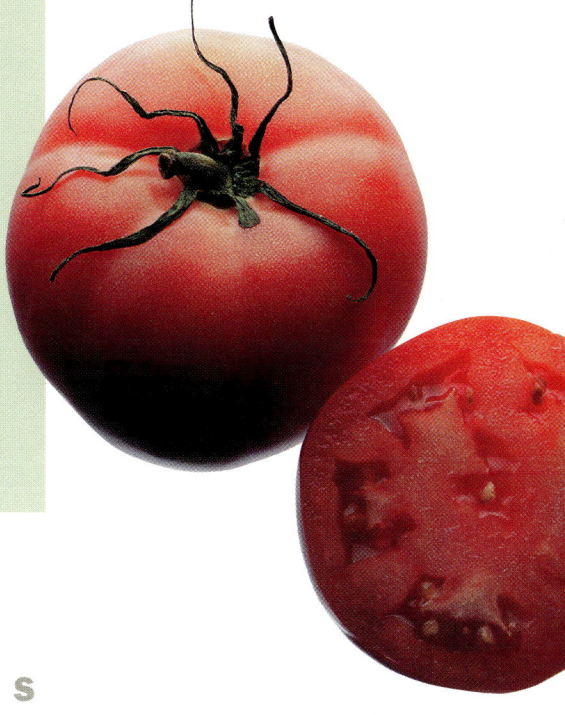

Tasty
HINTS

- For variations of the Quick Pizza Crust recipe, try adding seasonings such as oregano, basil, or thyme. You can also substitute 1 cup whole wheat flour, cornmeal, or other flour.

Helpful
HINTS

- To make these pizzas, you can either make your own crust using the recipe provided or you can purchase a prepared crust. Other options for quick crusts are frozen bread doughs, tortillas, French bread, pita bread, or Italian flat breads.

- For a crispy crust, bake the crust on a pizza stone or tile or on an inverted cookie sheet dusted with cornmeal.

- Make extra crusts to have ready for fast pizza dinners during the week. (Store the individual doughs in plastic wrap in the refrigerator for up to two days or in the freezer for up to two months. Bring to room temperature before using.)

- Vegetables such as broccoli and eggplant can be cooked before adding them to the pizza, if desired.

- For a thinner spread on the Mexican pizza, mix some of the salsa with the refried beans.

Mediterranean Pizza

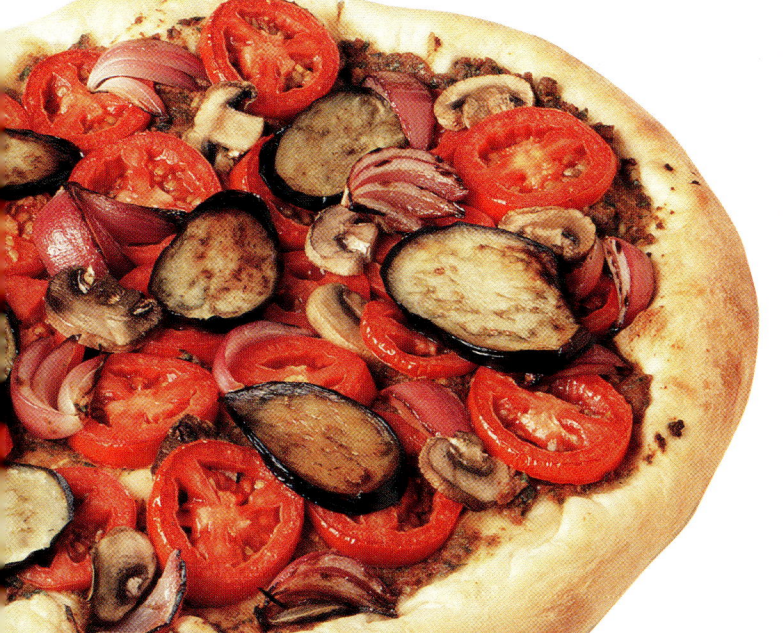

Pizza — Five International Variations

4 to 6 Servings

Cooking Directions for the Basic Recipe

1. Prepare crust. Preheat oven to 400 degrees.
2. Prepare spread.
3. Spray a large cookie sheet with a vegetable oil spray and place the crust(s) on the sheet.
4. Cover crust with the spread.
5. Add toppings and cheese, if used.
6. Bake at 400 degrees for approximately 12-15 minutes or until bubbly.

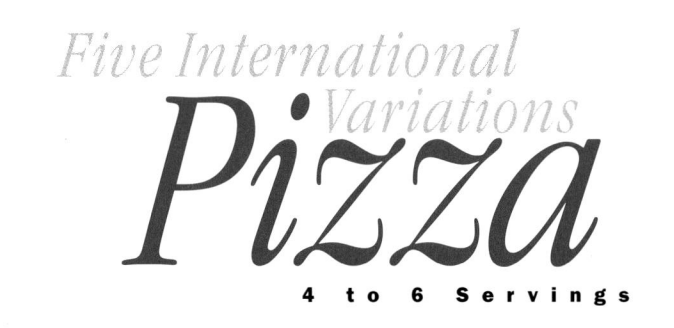

Ingredients	ASIAN	GREEK	ITALIAN	MEDITERRANEAN	MEXICAN
Crust	1 ready to use crust[h]	6 pita breads or 1 ready to use crust[h]	1 ready to use crust[h] or 1 large Italian flatbread	1 ready to use crust[h]	6 flour tortillas or 1 ready to use crust[h]
Spread	Mix the following together and then cook 2-3 minutes over medium heat: ¼ cup rice vinegar, ¼ cup pineapple juice (from tidbits), 2 T. soy sauce, 1 T. cornstarch, 1 tsp. garlic, minced, 1 tsp. fresh ginger, minced, ¼ tsp. pepper	Puree in blender: ½ cup raisins, 2 T. onion, chopped, ⅓ cup water	Cook the following over medium heat for 5 minutes: 16 oz. canned tomato sauce, 1 carrot, grated, 3 T. fresh basil, chopped, ½ tsp. oregano, ¼ tsp. pepper	Puree in blender: 1 T. olive oil, ⅓ cup water, 3 T. tomato paste, 1½ cups fresh basil, 3 cloves garlic, ¼ cup Romano or Parmesan cheese, 1 T. pine nuts or walnuts, salt	1 cup no-fat refried beans
Toppings	1 cup each, chopped: red pepper, broccoli; 1 cup water chestnuts, sliced; ½ cup pineapple tidbits; ½ cup bean sprouts	Chop finely in large bowl: 2 cups fresh spinach (tightly packed), 1 cup scallions. Add 1 T. pine nuts, 1 T. olive oil, ¼ cup lemon juice, ⅛ tsp. allspice, ⅛ tsp. pepper, salt	1 cup artichoke hearts, quartered; ½ cup thinly sliced sun-dried tomatoes*; 2 T. chopped black olives	1 cup each, thinly sliced: mushrooms or eggplant, plum tomatoes, red onion	½ cup each, diced: green chilies, onion; 1 cup plum tomatoes, sliced; 1 cup bell pepper, diced; 1 cup salsa
Cheese	½ cup firm tofu, crumbled	½ cup crumbled feta cheese, optional	½ cup mozzarella cheese, grated		½ cup cheddar cheese, grated

*Soaked in boiling water for 5 minutes and drained.
[h] See hints on the previous page.

Sauté

Helpful HINTS

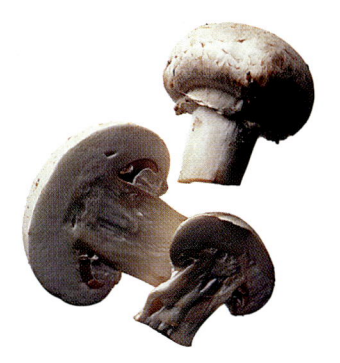

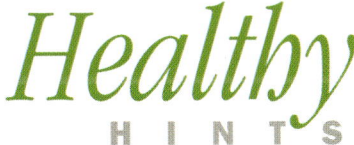

- In traditional sautéing, food is cooked in fat over high heat. However, you can also sauté food in small amounts of liquid such as broth, wine, juice, or even water. Add more of the liquid, if necessary, to keep the bottom of the pan moist as the liquid evaporates. To keep the vegetables from burning, cook over a medium-high heat and stir constantly. If you are cooking the food in oil, only a small amount is necessary – about a tablespoon for four servings. A non-stick skillet is helpful for cooking with minimal oil.

- Use fresh ginger root in these recipes. (Ground ginger is used primarily for baked items.) Fresh ginger can be stored in a plastic bag in the refrigerator for three weeks or in the freezer indefinitely.

Healthy HINTS

- Whole grains are higher in fiber, vitamin E, and several other vitamins and minerals.
- Brown rice has a chewier texture than white rice and is available in a quick cooking form.
- Basmati rice, commonly used in Indian cooking, has a nutlike fragrance and flavor. Couscous, a "pasta" popular in Northern Africa, is made from semolina wheat. Both are available in whole grain versions.

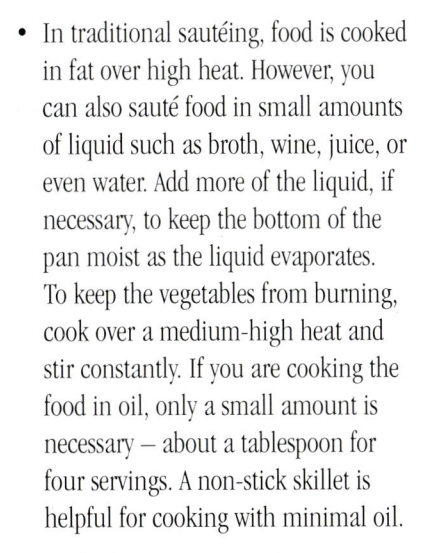

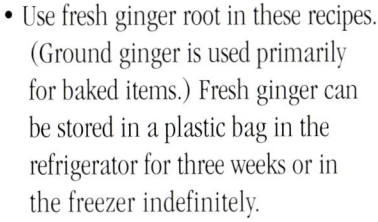

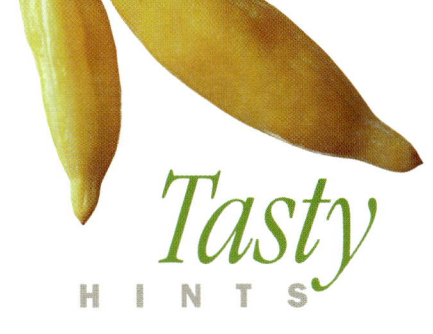

Tasty HINTS

- For added flavor, marinate the tofu in 2 T. soy sauce, 2 T. rice or cider vinegar, and 1 T. minced fresh ginger for at least 20 minutes.

- To enhance the flavor and aroma of the Indian spices, roast them first. Add the spices to a heavy preheated sauté pan and roast over low heat until they are light brown, shaking the pan or stirring to avoid burning. The spices can also be roasted in a small amount of oil.

- *To toast almonds*: Spread the nuts in a single layer on a baking sheet and toast in a 350° oven for 3-5 minutes or stir in a dry saucepan over low heat for 2-3 minutes. Watch them carefully so that they will be lightly toasted but not burned.

- For variety and added flavor and texture in the rice dishes:

    Try cooking another grain with the rice. For example, add some wheat berries, quinoa, barley, or wild rice.

    Cook the rice in other liquids such as broth, diluted juice, or flavored tea.

    For a richer, nuttier flavor, toast the grains in a dry pan over low heat for 10 minutes before cooking in the liquid.

- Try leftover grains for breakfast. Add juice or milk (low-fat, soy, or rice), raisins or other chopped fruit, and season with cinnamon and vanilla.

Five International Variations Sauté

4 to 6 Servings

Cooking Directions for the Basic Recipe

1. Begin cooking the grain.
2. Prepare all vegetables and seasonings.
3. Heat the sauté liquid in a large skillet. Add vegetables and seasonings. Cook on medium-high heat for 2-3 minutes.
4. Add the cooking liquid and the ad lib. Cook until all ingredients are at desired tenderness (3-7 minutes).
5. Serve vegetable mixture over cooked grain.

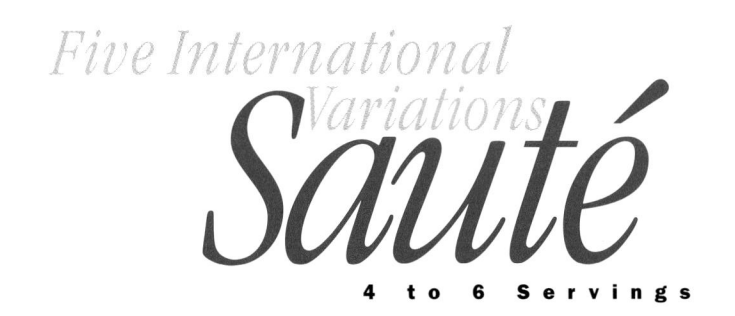

Ingredients	ASIAN	INDIAN	INDONESIAN	MEXICAN	MOROCCAN
Grain	1½ cup rice[g]	1½ cup basmati rice[g]	1½ cup rice[g]	1½ cup rice[g]	1½ cup couscous[g]
Vegetables	2 cups each: carrots, thinly sliced; broccoli, chopped; 3 cups mushrooms, sliced	2 cups carrots, finely diced; 1 cup each, diced: celery, apples, onions	1 cup each, chopped: onion, scallions; 2 cups green beans, trimmed and cut in 2" lengths; ¼ cup raisins	2 cups each, diced: onions, bell pepper; 1 cup tomatoes, chopped; 7 oz. can green chilies; ½ cup black olives, sliced	1 cup each, chopped: onion, cabbage; 2 cups each, chopped: tomato, bell pepper
Seasonings	1 T. fresh ginger, grated; 2 tsp. garlic, minced; ¼ tsp. pepper	1 tsp. ground cardamom[h]; 1 tsp. ground coriander; ¼ tsp. cinnamon; ⅛ tsp. ground cloves; ¼ tsp. ground cumin; ⅛ tsp. ground pepper (or 1 T. garam masala or curry powder)	1 T. garlic, minced; 1 T. curry powder; salt	2 tsp. garlic, minced; ½ tsp. chili powder; ½ cup fresh cilantro, chopped	½ tsp. cinnamon; ¼ tsp. nutmeg; ¼ tsp. pepper; salt; 2 T. raisins
Sauté Liquid	¼ cup broth	1 T. canola oil	Liquid from canned tomatoes	1 T. canola or olive oil	¼ cup white wine
Cooking Liquid	¼ cup orange juice; ¼ cup broth; 2 T. soy sauce; 1 T. rice vinegar; 2 tsp. sesame oil*	1 cup of broth	28 oz. can tomatoes, chopped	1 cup tomato juice	1 cup broth
Ad Lib[a]	8 oz. fish cut into small chunks (firm fish such as orange roughy, grouper, snapper) or 1 cup firm tofu[h], diced	2 T. slivered almonds, toasted[h]; 1 cup cooked garbanzo beans[g], optional	2 T. peanut butter	1 cup cooked black beans[g]	1 cup cooked chicken, diced

*To thicken the Asian cooking liquid: Mix 1 T. cornstarch with 2 T. cold water and stir in during last 2 minutes of cooking.

[h] See hints on the previous page.

[g] See guide on page 25.

[a] Use one of the suggested ingredients or substitute your own special ingredient.

Stir Fry

Healthy
HINTS

- Most deep green leafy vegetables are a good source of iron, calcium, folacin, and beta-carotene. Foods containing vitamin C, such as tomatoes or peppers, enhance the body's absorption of iron from plant foods.

- In the Indian version, coconut milk can be used in place of all or some of the milk. Although coconut milk is high in saturated fat, a small amount goes a long way in adding flavor and texture. Lower fat versions are also available.

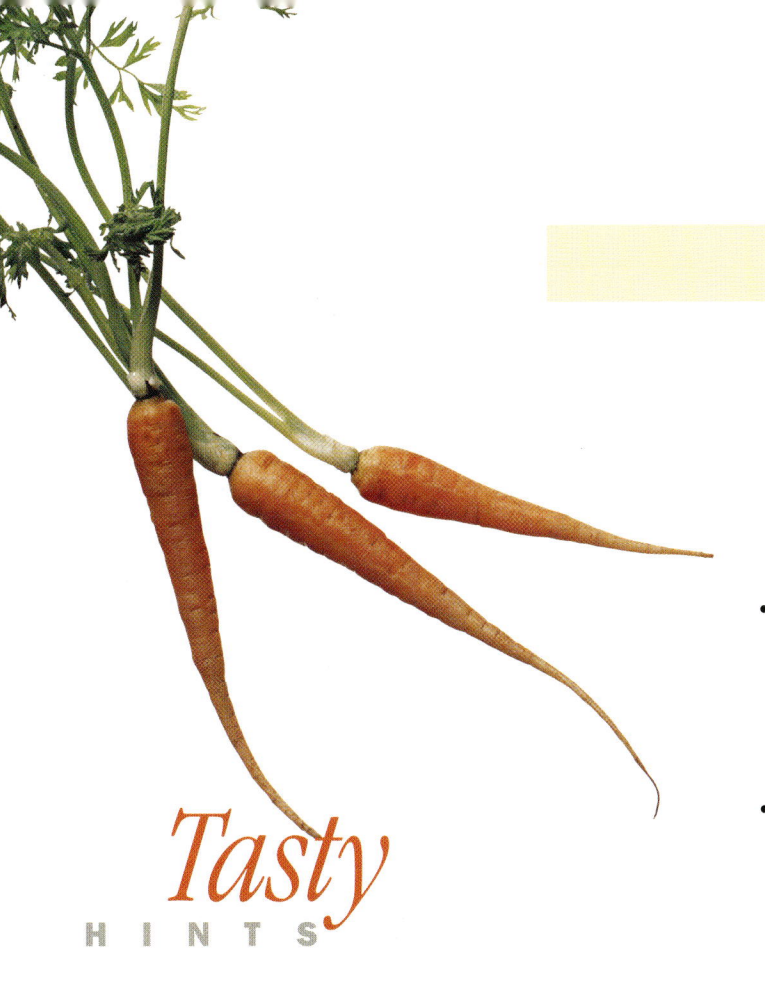

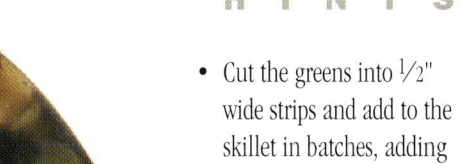

Tasty
HINTS

- For a variation, add chicken, fish, tofu or beans. For example, Asian – add chicken or tofu; Indian – add garbanzo beans; Mexican – add chicken or beans; Thai – add shrimp.

- Cut the fish or poultry into bite-sized pieces and cook in the oil for a few minutes. Remove from the pan while the vegetables are cooked, and return to the pan with the flavorings.

Helpful
HINTS

- Cut the greens into 1/2" wide strips and add to the skillet in batches, adding more as each batch wilts.

- Mirin is a sweet Japanese cooking wine made from rice. Sweet sherry can be substituted.

- Thai ingredients are available in many supermarkets and specialty shops.

Japanese Stir-Fry

Five International Variations *Stir Fry*

4 to 6 Servings

Cooking Directions for the Basic Recipe

1. Begin cooking the grain.
2. Prepare all vegetables.
3. Heat the oil in a skillet or wok. Add the seasonings and nuts and cook, stirring, for 20 seconds to 1 minute.
4. Add the vegetables and stir fry over high heat until vegetables are tender-crisp (3-7 minutes).
5. Stir in flavoring and heat.
6. Serve vegetables over the cooked grain.

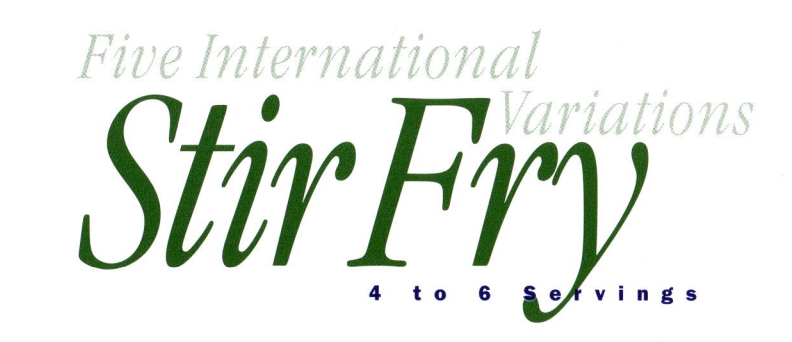

Ingredients	INDIAN	ITALIAN	JAPANESE	MEXICAN	THAI
Grain	1½ cup basmati rice[g]	12 oz. fettuccine[g]	12 oz. udon or soba noodles[g]	1½ cup rice[g]	1½ cups jasmine or other rice[g]
Vegetables	1 large bunch spinach, chopped 1 cup onion, diced 2 cups tomatoes, chopped	1 large bunch chard, chopped 2 cups broccoli, chopped 2 cup tomatoes, chopped	1 large bok choy, chopped 2 cups shitake or any mushrooms, sliced 1 cup red pepper strips	1 large bunch kale or collards, chopped 2 cups cauliflower, chopped 1 cup salsa	1 small head cabbage, chopped 2 cups celery, diced 1 cup carrot, grated
Oil	1 T. canola oil	1 T. olive oil	1 T. canola oil	1 T. canola oil	1 T. sesame oil
Seasonings	1 T. curry powder salt, optional	1 T. garlic, minced	1 T. fresh ginger, grated	1 T. chili powder 2 tsp. jalapeno pepper, minced	1 T. fresh ginger, minced ¼ tsp. Thai chili paste
Nuts	2 T. almonds	1 T. pine nuts optional	2 T. sesame seeds	2 T. walnuts, chopped or pine nuts	2 T. peanuts
Flavoring	¼ cup milk	⅓ cup Parmesan cheese 1 T. balsamic vinegar	1 tsp. sesame oil 1 T. mirin 1 T. soy sauce	1 cup fresh cilantro, chopped 1 T. lime juice	3 T. Thai fish sauce 2 T. lime juice

[g] See guide on page 25.

Oven Baked

Helpful
HINTS

- Although this meal takes a little longer to cook, the hands-on preparation time is less than 1/2 hour.

  Potatoes (white)
  Cook in boiling water for 15 minutes or until tender. Drain and set aside until ready to layer.

  To microwave: Cook sliced potatoes for 8 minutes. Although potatoes are not a grain, they are listed under this category for ease in following the recipe and because, like grains, they are rich in carbohydrates.

  Lentils
  Bring 1 1/2 cups of broth or water to a boil. Add 1/2 cup lentils and salt or seasonings if desired. Cover and simmer for 30 minutes or until tender. Cooking times for various kinds of lentils vary. 1/2 cup makes 1 1/2 cups cooked.

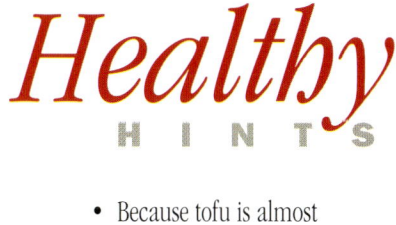

Healthy
HINTS

- Because tofu is almost tasteless and takes on the flavors of the foods it's cooked with, it is very versatile. A good source of protein, calcium, and iron, it has less saturated fat than cheese.

- Sweet potatoes are one of the most nutritious vegetables. They are rich in beta carotene and contain vitamin C, potassium, and fiber.

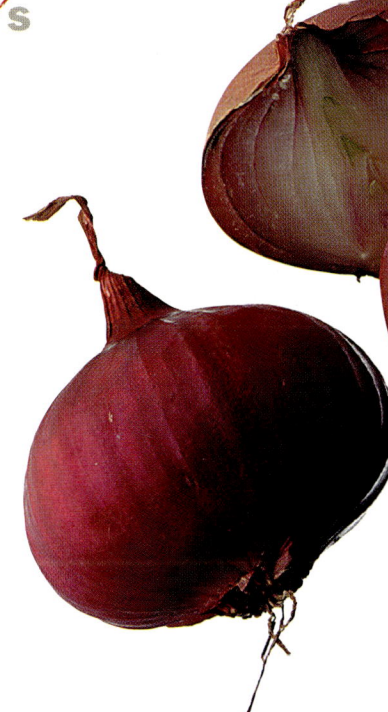

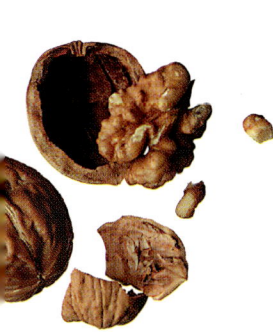

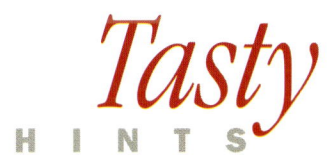

Tasty
HINTS

- 1 1/2 cups garbanzo beans (canned or cooked) can be substituted for the lentils.

- For a variation of the Indian version, puree the lentils or garbanzo beans in a blender or food processor.

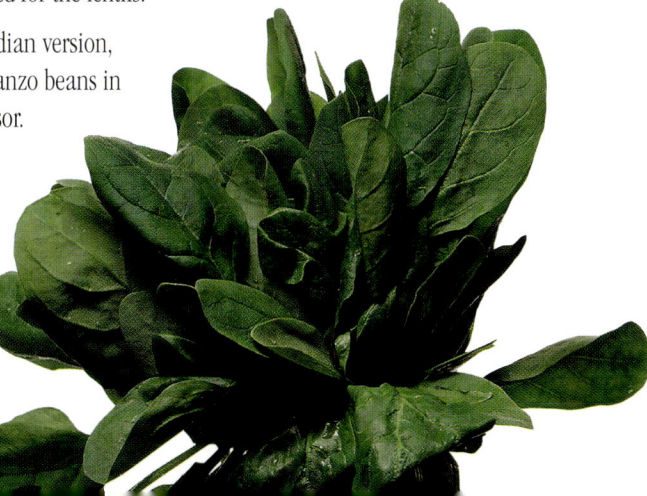

Five International Variations

Oven Baked

4 to 6 Servings

Cooking Directions for the Basic Recipe

1. Cook grain (except tortillas) and lentils (if using in the Indian version).
2. Prepare vegetables and seasonings.
3. Heat sauté liquid. Add vegetables and cook over medium-high heat for 5 minutes.
4. Add seasonings and cook an additional 3 minutes.
5. In a 9" by 13" casserole dish coated lightly with vegetable oil, layer ½ (each): grain, vegetable mixture, and ad lib. Repeat. Drizzle liquid over top, if used.
6. Cover and bake at 400 degrees for 35-45 minutes.

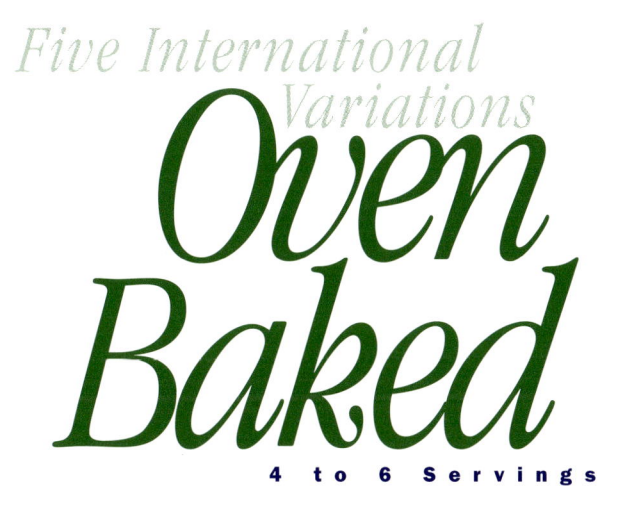

Ingredients	FRENCH	INDIAN	ITALIAN	MEDITERRANEAN	MEXICAN
Grain	3 medium baking potatoes[h], sliced ⅛" thick	1½ cups basmati rice[g]	8 oz. lasagna noodles[g]	1½ cups polenta*[g]	12 corn tortillas
Vegetables	1 cup onion, chopped 3 cups zucchini, chopped 3 cups tomatoes, chopped	1 cup onions, diced 2 sweet potatoes, grated 2 cups carrots, grated 16 oz. can tomato sauce	1 cup each, chopped: scallions, green peppers 2 cups each, thinly sliced: mushrooms, zucchini 43 oz. canned crushed tomatoes	20 oz. frozen spinach (thawed and drained) 3 cups tomatoes, chopped 2 cups mushrooms, sliced ¼ cup sliced black olives	1 cup each, diced: onion, bell pepper, tomatoes 1 cup corn 1 cup salsa
Seasonings	2 tsp. tarragon 1 T. fresh parsley, chopped ¼ tsp. pepper salt	1 T. fresh ginger, minced 1 T. garlic, minced 1 tsp. cumin 1 tsp. turmeric ½ tsp. cinnamon ½ tsp. ground coriander salt	1 tsp. garlic, minced 2 tsp. basil 2 tsp. oregano ¼ tsp. pepper salt	2 tsp. garlic, minced ¾ tsp. thyme ¾ tsp. oregano ¼ tsp. pepper salt	2 tsp. garlic, minced 1 tsp. chili powder
Sauté Liquid	2 tsp. olive oil or ¼ cup broth	2 tsp. olive or canola oil	2 tsp. olive oil or ¼ cup broth	2 tsp. olive oil or ¼ cup broth	2 tsp. canola oil or ¼ cup broth
Ad Lib[a]	¾ cup Parmesan cheese	1½ cups cooked lentils[h]	12 oz. firm tofu, mashed and ½ cup parmesan cheese or 16 oz. tofu, mashed	5 oz. feta cheese, crumbled or mozzarella cheese, grated	¾ cup low fat Cheddar or Monterey Jack cheese
Drizzle Liquid	⅓ cup white wine mixed with 2 T. Worcestershire sauce and 2 T. flour	3 T. lemon juice mixed with 1 T. olive or canola oil	Use some of the vegetable mixture for the top layer		⅓ cup broth

*Cooked in 3 cups of water and 3 cups broth.

[h] See hints on the previous page.

[g] See guide on page 25.

[a] Use one of the suggested ingredients or substitute your own special ingredient.

Soup

Healthy HINTS

- Soups are a delicious and easy way to get some of the 3-5 daily servings of vegetables recommended for good health.
- Pureeing all or part of the soup gives it a "creamy" texture without adding extra fat. Soups can also be thickened by adding a starch such as rice or potato or by adding evaporated skim milk.
- You can use a low-sodium broth to lessen the salt content and adjust the seasonings to your taste.

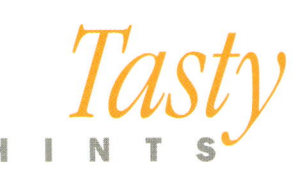

Tasty HINTS

- The longer the soups cook, the more the flavors will blend and intensify.
- Add rice, noodles or beans for a heartier version of the vegetable soup.
- Serve any of the soups with a crusty bread and salad for a complete meal.

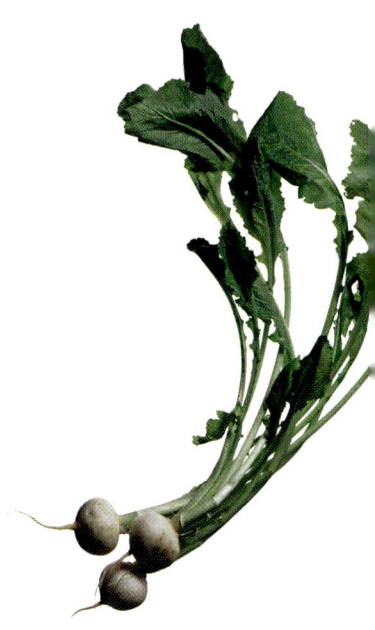

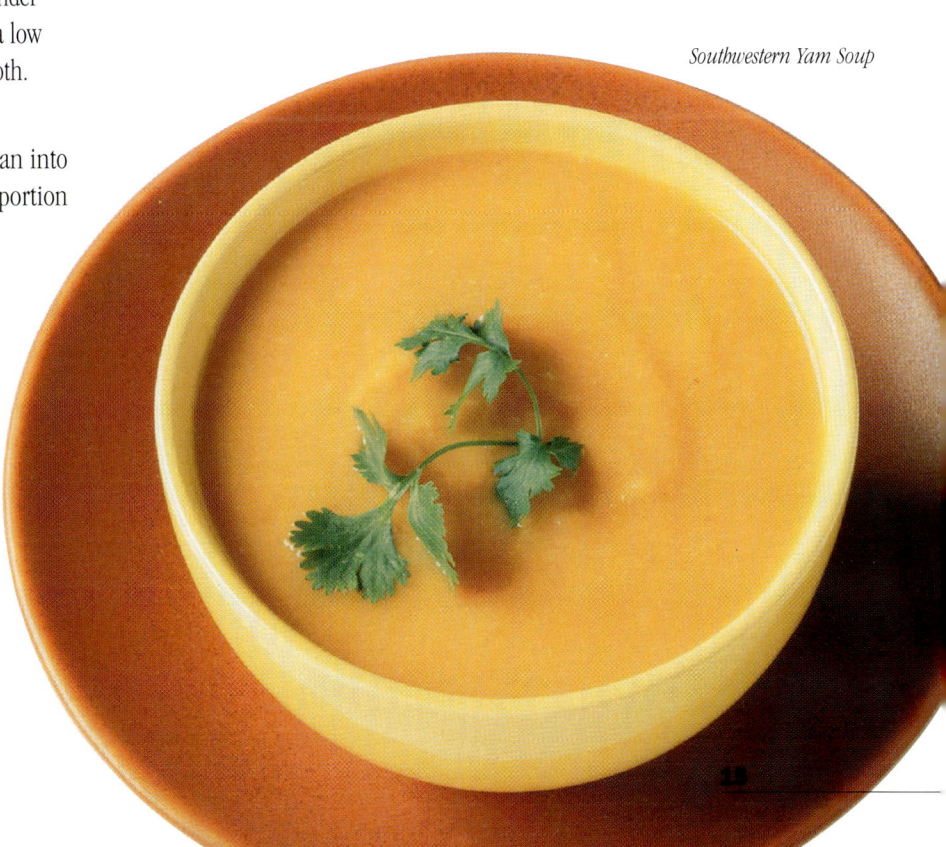

Helpful HINTS

- *To puree*: It's best to puree the soup in batches. Fill a blender about $1/3$ full, wrap a dishtowel around the lid, start on a low speed and gradually increase the speed. Puree until smooth. You can also use a food processor.
- *Partial puree*: Pour half of the soup from your saucepan into a blender and puree until smooth. Return the pureed portion to the saucepan and stir.
- *To toast the bread:* Cut or tear a loaf of bread into small pieces. Toast in a 350° oven for 5-8 minutes until the bread is dry. Breadcrumbs may be substituted, if desired.
- Chop the vegetables into small pieces so they'll cook quickly. Add vegetables that take longer to cook, such as sweet potatoes and carrots, before adding quicker cooking vegetables such as tomatoes.

Southwestern Yam Soup

Five International Variations Soup
6 to 8 Servings

Cooking Directions for the Basic Recipe

1. Heat oil in large (at least 4 qt.) saucepan.
2. Add vegetables and cook for about 5 minutes over medium/medium high heat.
3. Add liquid, legumes if used, and seasonings.
4. Simmer, covered, for 20 minutes over low heat* or until vegetables and legumes are cooked.

   *For the Southwestern Yam soup, cook over medium heat for 20 minutes or until the yams are soft.
5. Puree[h] all or part of the soup according to chart below.

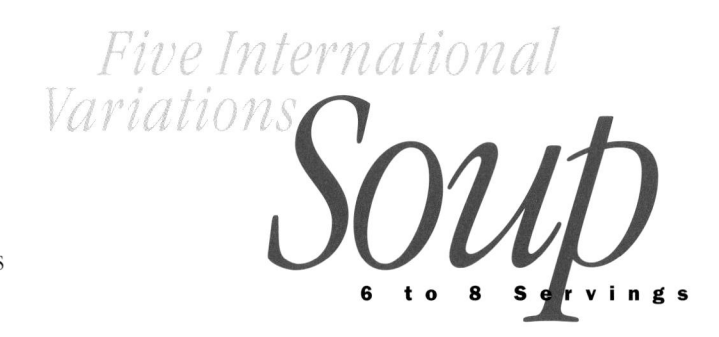

Ingredients	CALIFORNIAN Vegetable	INDIAN Curried Lentil	MEDITERRANEAN Onion	MIDDLE EASTERN Hummus	SOUTHWESTERN Yam
Oil	1 T. olive oil	1 T. olive oil	1 T. olive oil	1 T. olive oil	1 T. canola or olive oil
Vegetables	1 cup onion, finely chopped 2 T. garlic, minced ½ cup carrot, finely chopped 1 cup zucchini, finely chopped ½ cup celery, chopped 1 14 oz. can diced tomatoes or 5 plum tomatoes, diced ¼ cup tomato paste	1 cup onion, chopped ¼ cup carrots, finely chopped ¼ cup celery, chopped 2 T. fresh garlic, minced	5 cups onions, thinly sliced 2 T. garlic, minced	1 cup onion, chopped 4 T. garlic, minced ½ cup carrot, finely chopped 1 cup celery, chopped	4 medium yams, diced 1 cup onions, chopped 2 T. fresh garlic, minced ¼ cup carrots, finely chopped ¼ cup celery, chopped
Liquid	6 cups broth[g]	8 cups broth[g]	7 cups broth[g]	1½ T. lemon juice 5 cups broth[g]	4 cups broth[g] plus 2 cups water
Legumes		1 cup red lentils, uncooked		2½ cups cooked garbanzo beans	
Seasonings	1 T. oregano ½ T. basil ¼ tsp. pepper salt to taste	2 tsp. turmeric 2 tsp. curry 1 T. plus 1 tsp. fresh ginger, minced ¼ tsp. pepper salt to taste	4 T. parsley, chopped 3 T. parmesan ½ tsp. pepper salt to taste 2 cups bread, cut into small pieces and toasted[h]	1 T. tahini 3 T. fresh ginger, minced 1 tsp. cumin ¼ tsp. pepper salt to taste 2 T. parsley, chopped (optional garnish)	⅛ tsp. cayenne pepper ¼ tsp. sage ¼ tsp. cumin ¼ tsp. pepper salt to taste
Puree[h]	none	all	Partial	all	all

[h] See hints on the previous page
[g] See guide on page 25

Healthy Grains
HINTS

- Choose whole grains such as brown rice, whole-wheat couscous, and whole grain breads whenever possible. These are richer in nutrients and fiber than their more processed counterparts. Although they take longer to cook, the added nutrients, texture, and flavor make them worth the additional preparation time. Quick-cooking brown rice is available.

- Quinoa (KEEN-wa) is technically not a grain but cooks like one. It is a complete protein, which is unusual for a plant food. It is almost gluten-free, making it a good alternative for people with allergies to wheat. Its nutty flavor is highlighted in the Southwestern recipe by the addition of pecans and walnuts.

- Most of the fat in nuts is not saturated. In fact, they're a good source of beneficial fats. Nuts also contain fiber, protein, vitamins and minerals. You can include them in moderate amounts in a healthy diet. Toasting nuts gives them a rich flavor so you can use a smaller amount.

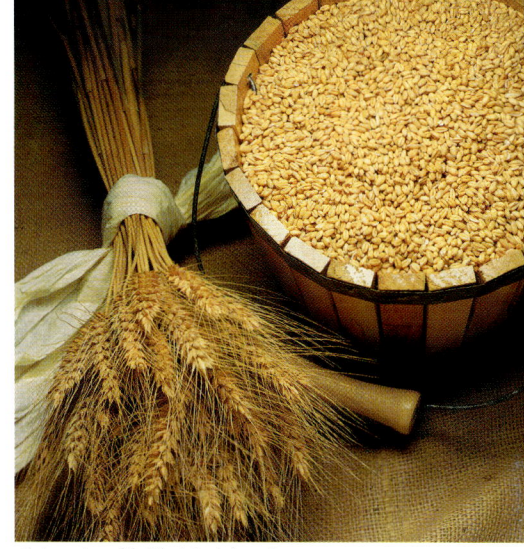

Photo courtesy of the Wheat Foods Council

Helpful HINTS

- Cooking times:
  White rice: 20 minutes; *Brown rice:* 45 minutes; *Quinoa*: 15-20 minutes; *Couscous*: add the liquid, stir, and remove from heat; *Whole wheat Couscous:* simmer 5 minutes, let sit 10 minutes.

- Cook extra rice and use it to make another quick meal. The next day, you can re-heat the rice, add more vegetables, fish, chicken, or tofu and make a stir-fry!

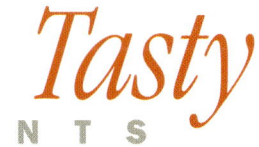

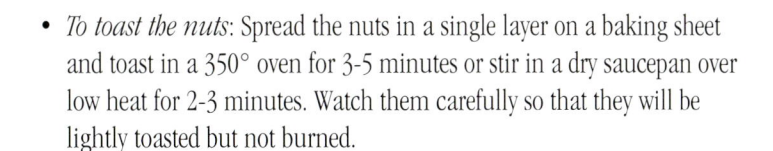

Tasty HINTS

- *To toast the nuts*: Spread the nuts in a single layer on a baking sheet and toast in a 350° oven for 3-5 minutes or stir in a dry saucepan over low heat for 2-3 minutes. Watch them carefully so that they will be lightly toasted but not burned.

- Try some of the aromatic rices for variety – basmati, texmati, and jasmine. Cook them as you would regular rice.

- Wild rice blends offer another flavor option. Wild rice is actually the seed of a grass and has a strong flavor and chewy texture that goes well with brown rice or barley. These blends usually require about 45 minutes of cooking.

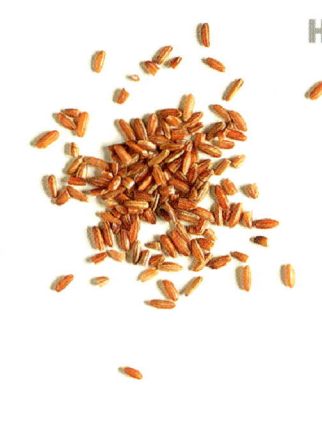

Five International Variations
Grains
4 to 6 Servings

Cooking Directions for the Basic Recipe

1. Heat the oil in a large saucepan.
2. Add the vegetables and cook for 2-3 minutes over medium heat.
3. Add the seasonings and grain, cook for another 2 minutes.
4. Add the liquid and bring to a boil. Reduce heat and simmer, covered, until the grain is cooked. See previous tips page for cooking times.
5. Add the toppings and blend all together (let the black beans heat through) before serving.

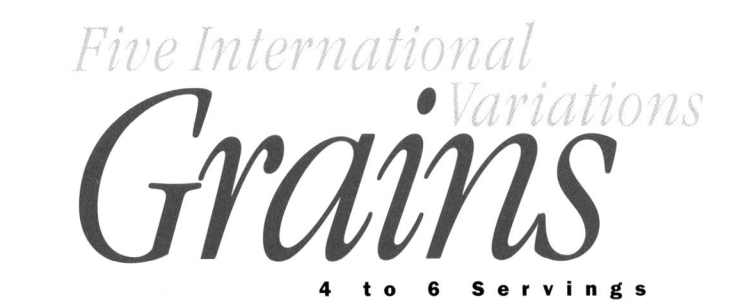

Ingredients	ASIAN Rice	ITALIAN Rice	MEXICAN Rice	MOROCCAN Conscous	SOUTHWESTERN Quinoa
Oil*	1 T. canola or olive oil	1 T. olive oil	1 T. olive oil	1 T. olive oil	1 T. canola oil or olive oil
Vegetables	1 cup onions, chopped ½ cup carrots, grated	¾ cup onion, chopped ¼ cup sun-dried tomatoes** (rehydrated and finely chopped)	1½ cups onion, chopped	¾ cup red onion, chopped	1 cup onion, minced
Seasonings	1 T. fresh ginger, minced ¼ tsp. pepper salt to taste	2 tsp. garlic, minced 1 T. basil ¼ tsp. pepper salt to taste	1½ T. garlic, minced ¾ tsp. cumin ¼ tsp. pepper salt to taste	1½ tsp. fresh garlic, minced ½ tsp. cinnamon 1½ T. fresh marjoram, chopped 2 T. raisins ¼ tsp. pepper salt to taste	1 T. garlic, minced 1½ tsp. ground coriander ½ tsp. pepper salt to taste
Grain	1¼ cups rice[h]	1¼ cups rice[h]	1¼ cups rice[h]	1¼ cups couscous[h]	1¼ cups quinoa[†]
Liquid	2½ cups broth[g] 1½ tsp. sesame oil 1½ tsp. soy sauce	2 cups water Juice of 1 orange (about ½ cup)	2½ cups broth[g] 1 cup cooked black beans	¾ cup tomato juice ¾ cup water	2½ cups broth[g]
Topping	2 T. scallions, chopped (optional garnish)	2 T. pine nuts, toasted[h]	3 T. fresh cilantro, chopped	2 T. slivered almonds, toasted[h]	2 T. walnut pieces, toasted[h] 2 T. pecans, toasted[h]

*Broth or other liquid can be substituted for the oil.

**Soaked in boiling water for 5 minutes and drained.

[g] See guide on page 25.

[h] See hints on the previous page.

[†] Rinse and drain the quinoa first to remove a bitter residue that sometimes remains on the seeds.

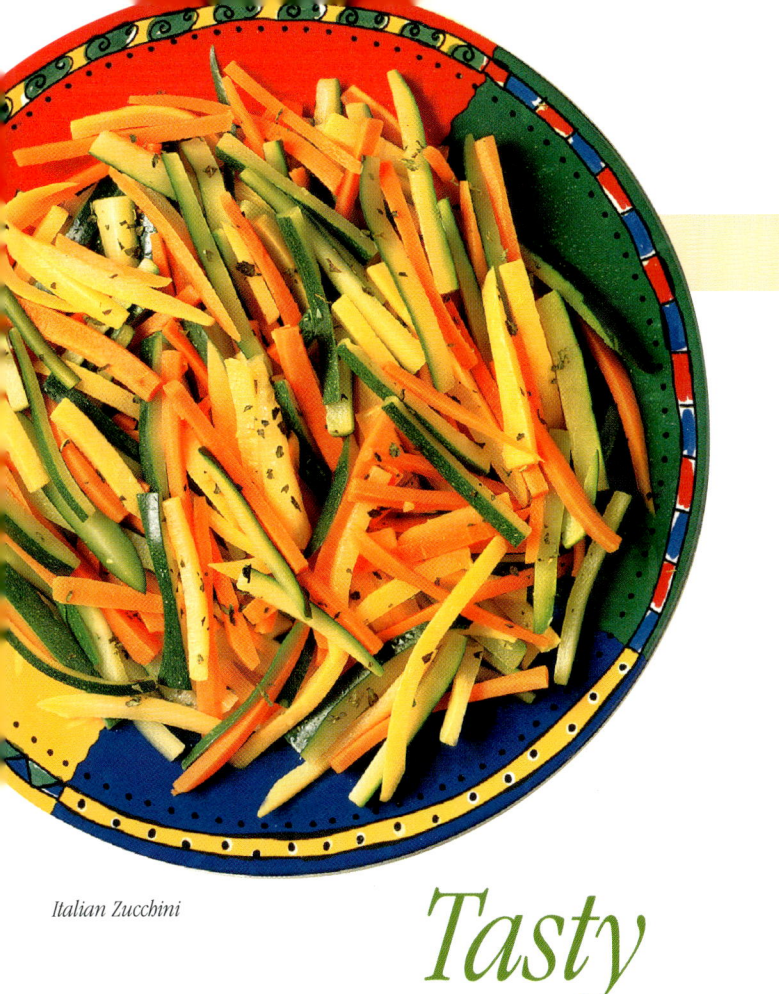

Veggies

Italian Zucchini

Helpful HINTS

- Nothing beats the flavor of fresh vegetables. Other convenient, timesaving options include frozen, canned, pre-cut packaged, and salad bar vegetables.

- You can turn the Mexican Peppers and Onions into fajitas. On a large tortilla, spoon some of the cooked vegetables; fresh chopped tomatoes; shredded lettuce; cheese or cooked, shredded chicken; and salsa.

- You can also steam or microwave the vegetables first. Meanwhile, combine the liquid (omit the water from the carrot and broccoli recipes) and seasonings. Pour the seasoning mixture over the vegetables.

Tasty HINTS

- If vegetables are not one of your favorite foods, keep trying different ones. With the wide variety of colors, flavors and textures to choose from, you're sure to find some you like. Try them raw or cooked.

- Use vegetables that are in season whenever possible.

- *To steam vegetables:* Cut vegetables into chunks and place in a metal steamer. Place the steamer into a pot that has about an inch of boiling water in it. Add vegetables, cover the pot and adjust the heat to keep the water simmering. Cook until the vegetables are cooked to desired tenderness, adding additional water if necessary.

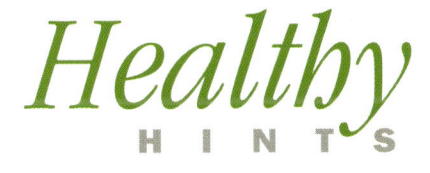

Healthy HINTS

- Eat a wide variety of deeper-colored vegetables and fruit. In general, these have the most nutrients. Beneficial plant substances called phytochemicals are what give plants their rich color and flavor.

- When shopping for vegetables, buy 3 different colors for variety in flavor and nutrients.

- Eat a minimum of five servings of fruits and vegetables each day for optimal health. Most people underestimate the amount to buy. For example, if there are 4 people in your family and you shop for 5 days of groceries, you'll need to buy 100 servings! A serving is $1/2$ cup of cooked vegetables, 1 cup leafy vegetables, or 1 medium fruit.

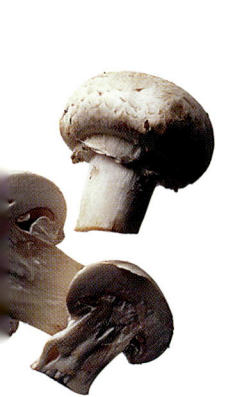

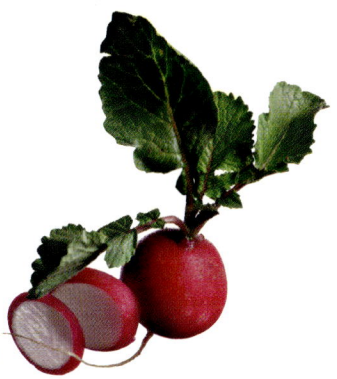

Cooking Directions for the Basic Recipe

1. Add all the liquid and seasonings to a large saucepan, stir together and heat.
2. Add the vegetables and cook on medium heat until the vegetables are cooked to desired tenderness. (About 5-10 minutes for all except the carrots which take 15-20 minutes)

If the vegetables begin to stick to the bottom of the pan as you cook them, add a little more water. See previous cooking tips page for more vegetable cooking options.

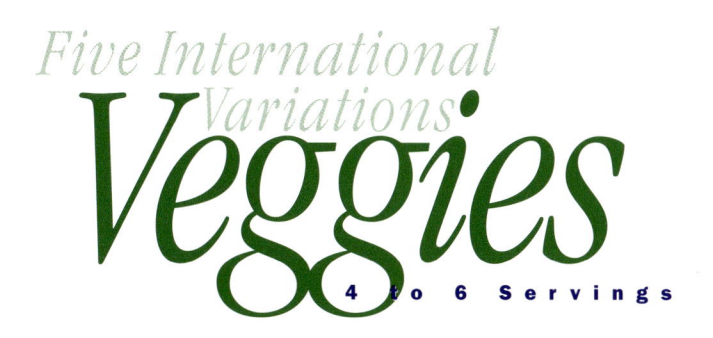

Five International Variations
Veggies
4 to 6 Servings

Ingredients	ASIAN Carrots	FRENCH Broccoli	ITALIAN Zucchini	MEXICAN Peppers & Onions	IRISH Green Beans
Liquid	2 tsp. canola oil or olive oil 1 tsp. sesame oil ¼ cup water*	1 T. fresh lemon juice ½ cup water	2 tsp. olive oil 1 tsp. red wine vinegar	1 T. olive oil juice of 1 lime	½ cup malt vinegar**
Seasonings	2 tsp. fresh ginger, minced 1 T. sesame seeds, toasted 2 tsp. fresh cilantro, chopped, optional ⅛ tsp. pepper salt to taste	2 T. almonds, crushed 3 T. fresh parsley, finely chopped 1½ tsp. lemon zest ¼ tsp. pepper salt to taste	½ T. garlic, minced 1 tsp. oregano 1 tsp. basil salt and pepper to taste	½ tsp. chili powder 2-3 tsp. cumin salt to taste	1½-2 T. brown sugar salt and pepper to taste
Vegetables	8 large carrots, chopped ½ cup chopped scallions	4½ cups broccoli	2 green zucchini* 2 yellow zucchini squash* 1 carrot* *cut all into 2 inch chunks and then into thin ¼ inch strips	2 red peppers, thinly sliced 2 green peppers, thinly sliced 1 onion, thinly sliced	5 cups green beans, trimmed and cut into 2" lengths (or substitute 1 small head of cabbage)

* 2 T. of orange juice can be substituted for 2 T. of water.
** For a sweeter flavor, you can use balsamic vinegar.

Chicken Fish & Soy

Tasty HINTS

- Dry marinades or rubs (as in the Cajun chicken recipe) are an easy way to add flavor. The mixture of herbs and spices can be made in large quantities and stored in jars for later use.

Helpful HINTS

- Pat the tofu dry with paper towels before marinating to allow more of the marinade to be absorbed.
- For an attractive presentation, slice the cooked chicken into thin slices and fan it on the plate. Cut the tofu in half diagonally and then in half a second time, again diagonally. Serve over rice.
- Instead of baking or grilling, cut the marinated food into pieces and sauté in a pan with assorted, chopped vegetables. Serve over rice or noodles.
- *Bake*: Chicken – 350°, approximately 20-30 minutes, until the chicken if firm and fully cooked. Fish – 450°, about 10 minutes per inch of thickness at thickest part, or until fish is just opaque and flakes when tested with a fork. Soy – 350°, about 15 minutes. Optional: broil the chicken, fish, or soy for a minute or two at the end of baking to brown.
- *Grill*: About 3-10 minutes on each side. Use any extra marinade to baste the food as it cooks on the grill. If grilling the Cajun chicken, brush lightly with olive oil before cooking.

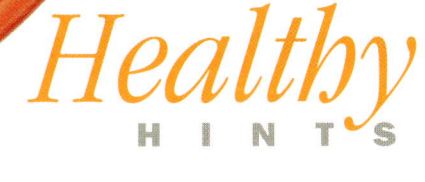

Asian Tofu and Rice

Healthy HINTS

- Instead of having meat or chicken at the center of the plate, use them more as a condiment with serving sizes of about three ounces (3 ounces is the size of a deck of cards). Serve with larger amounts of grains and vegetables.
- Fish and poultry are good choices since they are low in saturated fat. Fish, particularly fattier fish such as salmon and tuna, contain a beneficial type of unsaturated fat called omega 3 fatty acids.
- Most of the fat in tofu and other soy products is unsaturated. The soybean is a complete protein since it contains all the essential amino acids.
- Diversify your protein intake by including more plant sources – beans, grains, and nuts and seeds. These foods are also a good source of fiber and other nutrients.

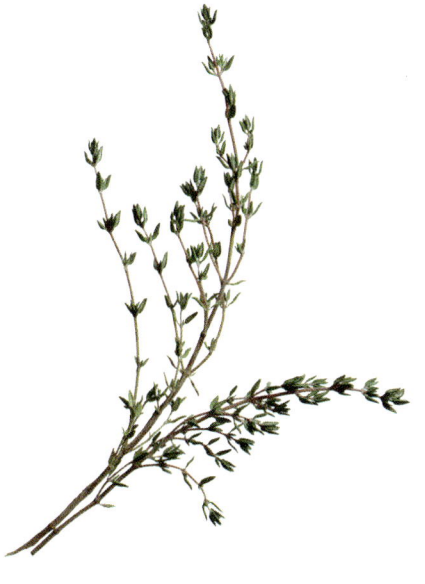

Five International Variations
Chicken Fish & Soy
4 to 5 Servings

Cooking Directions for the Basic Recipe

1. Mix marinade together in a bowl.
2. Place the fish, chicken, or tofu in a baking dish and cover it with the marinade. Turn to coat. For more flavor, let it marinate for at least 20 minutes, refrigerated, turning it from time to time.
3. Spray a baking dish with cooking oil or brush lightly with oil. Bake or grill until cooked. Test for doneness. See baking hints on the previous page.
4. Cut into individual serving sizes[h] and serve with vegetables and/or salad and a grain.

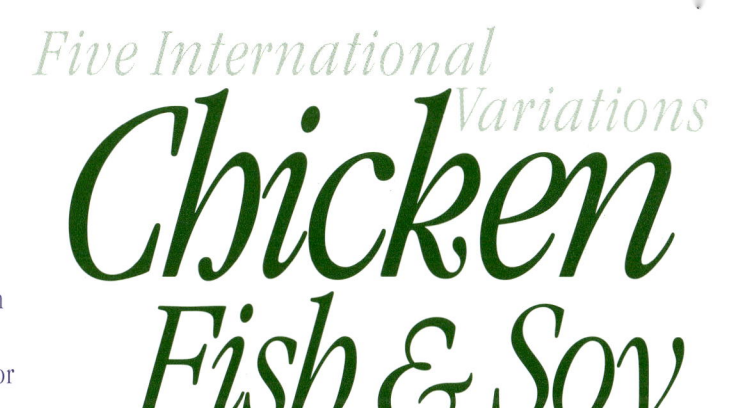

Ingredients	ASIAN Tofu	CAJUN Chicken	CUBAN Fish	FRENCH Salmon	MEDITERRANEAN Chicken
Marinade	2 T. soy sauce[g] 1-2 T. sesame oil 1 tsp. fresh garlic, minced 2 tsp. brown sugar or orange juice 1 tsp. fresh ginger, minced ⅛ tsp. cayenne pepper	1 T. paprika 1 tsp. thyme 1 tsp. oregano ½ tsp. garlic powder ⅛ tsp. cayenne pepper ½ tsp. salt	¼ cup fresh lime juice (juice of 2 limes) ½ T. olive oil ½ T. fresh garlic, minced 2 T. fresh oregano, chopped or 2 tsp. dried ⅛ tsp. pepper pinch salt pinch cumin	3 T. white wine 2 tsp. dill 1 tsp. garlic powder or fresh minced ⅛ tsp. pepper 1 lemon, thinly sliced (arrange lemon slices over fish before cooking and use as garnish)	2 T. balsamic vinegar 2 tsp. dijon mustard ½ T. olive oil 1 T. fresh garlic, minced ½ tsp. oregano ¼ tsp. pepper
Chicken, Fish or Soy	1 lb. firm or extra firm tofu[h], cut in half horizontally, pressed to remove extra water	1 lb. boneless, skinless chicken	1 lb. halibut or any firm white fish	1 lb. salmon	1 lb. skinless, boneless chicken

[h] See hints on the previous page

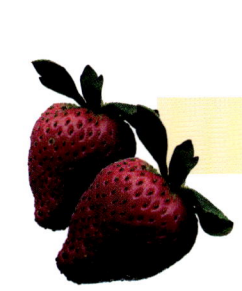

Dessert

Tasty HINTS

- Each dessert recipe can be served fresh, cooked, or with other foods. Serve the fruit mixture over: yogurt, frozen yogurt or low-fat ice cream, sorbet, cereal, pancakes, waffles and muffins.

- Or wrap the fruit mixture in phyllo dough and bake in a 350° oven for about 10 minutes.

Healthy HINTS

- Enjoy these fruit dishes as snacks as well as desserts. They're a delicious and easy way to get some of the recommended 2-4 daily servings of fruits, while satisfying a sweet tooth.

- Fruits are a good source of beneficial antioxidants and phytochemicals.

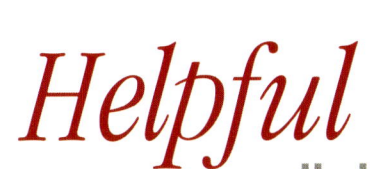

Helpful HINTS

- Make your dessert first, before cooking dinner. This will allow all the flavors to blend and increases the flavor.

- Feel free to adjust the proportions of fruits, as well as the types of fruits used. Take advantage of seasonal fruits and whatever you have on hand. For example, try mango with pineapple or strawberries with bananas.

- In the French Citrus Supreme recipe, strain the raspberry mixture to remove the seeds if you would like a smoother texture.

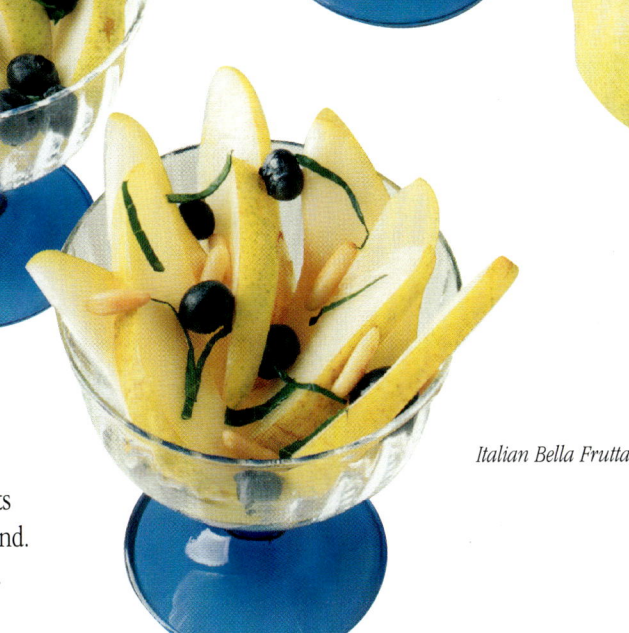

Italian Bella Frutta

Five International Variations
Dessert
4 to 6 Servings

Cooking Directions for the Basic Recipe

1. Slice or chop the fruit and place into a large bowl.
2. Mix the liquid and seasonings together in a small bowl.
3. Pour the liquid mixture over the fruit.

   Optional: Place fruit mixture in saucepan and heat on medium heat for a few minutes. For a thicker sauce, add 1 tsp. of cornstarch mixed with a little water.
4. Sprinkle toppings over the fruit mixture.

*Depending on the ripeness of fruit, you may need to add a little honey or other sweetener.

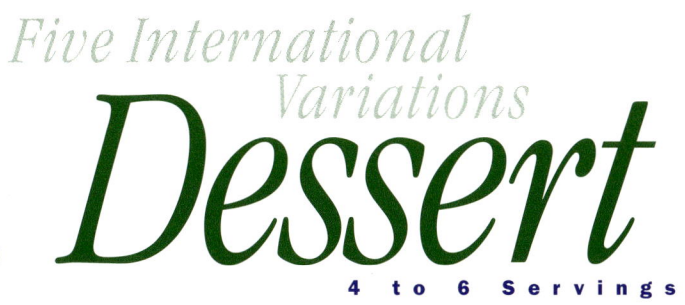

Ingredients	HAWAIIAN Medley	ITALIAN Bella Frutta	FRENCH Citrus Supreme	AMERICAN Apple Berry	NEW ZEALAND Delight
Fruits	4 bananas, sliced 1 cup pineapple chunks 3 T. raisins	3 pears, sliced 1 cup blueberries, fresh or frozen	3 oranges, peeled and sliced	3 apples, chopped 1½ cups blackberries, fresh or frozen	2½ cups fresh strawberries, sliced 5 kiwi, sliced
Liquid	3 T. pineapple juice	2½ T. apple juice concentrate	Puree in a blender: 1 T. orange juice 1½ cups fresh or frozen raspberries 1 tsp. honey	½ cup apple juice concentrate 3 T. vanilla yogurt	¼ cup lemon sorbet, juice of ½ orange (about 3 T.)
Seasonings	¼ tsp. allspice	½ tsp. almond flavoring 2 tsp. fresh basil, very finely shredded ⅛ tsp. nutmeg		¼ tsp. cinnamon	¼ tsp. dry ginger
Toppings	1 T. unsalted peanuts, crushed	1 T. pine nuts, toasted*	1 T. pecans, toasted*	1 T. walnut pieces, toasted*	1 T. sliced almonds, toasted*

*Toasting nuts – see hints on page 17.
Crunchy nut cereal can be used instead of the nuts, if desired.

A Guide to Ingredients

Reducing Salt and Fat

Beans - In all the recipes calling for cooked beans, canned beans can be used as a convenient alternative to dried beans.

To reduce the amount of sodium in canned beans, drain and rinse or buy low-sodium varieties.

Broth - use vegetable or chicken broth (either homemade, canned, powder, or cubes) in any recipe calling for broth. If you want to reduce sodium, try one of the reduced-sodium or sodium-free products available.

Cheese - you can reduce the amount of fat, saturated fat, and calories in a recipe by using less cheese or by using a reduced-fat version. Tofu and soy cheeses are lower in saturated fat and offer another flavor option. Reduced-fat versions are available.

Soy sauce - use reduced-sodium versions of soy sauce or tamari for 35-40% less sodium.

Oils - use flavorful oils such as dark (Asian) sesame oil and extra-virgin olive oil. This allows you to use small amounts and still enjoy a rich flavor.

Adding Flavor

When lemon or lime juice is an ingredient, fresh juice is recommended since it adds a much better flavor than bottled juices.

Some of these recipes include wine as an ingredient. Most of the alcohol evaporates during the cooking process, leaving the flavor of the wine. Broth can be substituted for wine in all of these recipes.

To ensure that all vegetables are cooked to the desired tenderness, you can add those that require more cooking first and the quicker cooking vegetables a couple of minutes later.

Measurements

Herbs and spices - amounts given are for dried herbs and spices unless fresh herbs are specified. When substituting dried herbs for fresh ones, use approximately ¼ the amount.

Salt - specific amounts are not given so that you can vary the amounts to your individual preferences.

The following uncooked ingredients, chopped, equal one cup.

Apple	1 medium
Bell pepper	1 medium
Cabbage	⅕ small head
Carrot	2 large
Celery	2 medium stalks
Cucumber	½ medium
Green beans	⅓ lb
Mushrooms	4 oz
Onion	1 medium
Scallions	5 onions
Tomato	1 medium (or 3 plum)
Zucchini	1 small
Hard cheese, shredded	4 oz
Parmesan, grated	3 oz

1 medium clove garlic = 1 tsp., minced
14 oz. canned tomatoes = 2 cups chopped fresh tomatoes

Cooking Grains

The "grain" amount in all of these recipes refers to the uncooked amount.

Rice: In a saucepan, bring to a boil two cups of liquid for each cup of rice. Add salt or seasonings, if used. Slowly stir in the rice, cover, and cook over low heat until all the liquid is absorbed.
20 minutes for white rice
45 minutes for brown rice
Fluff with fork. 1 cup makes 3 cups cooked.

Couscous: Bring 1½ cups water or broth to a boil for each cup of couscous. Add salt or seasonings, if desired. Add couscous, stir, and remove from heat. Cover and let stand 5 minutes. Fluff with fork. 1 cup makes 2½ cups cooked.

Polenta (coarse ground cornmeal): In a large pot, bring to a boil 4 cups of liquid for each cup of corn meal. Stir in the corn meal gradually and stir for about three minutes until the mixture thickens. Add salt or seasonings, if used. Reduce heat and simmer, stirring often, for 15 - 20 minutes or until mixture pulls away from sides of saucepan. One cup makes 3½ cups.

Pasta/Noodles: Gradually add 1 pound of pasta to 5 quarts of rapidly boiling water. Cook uncovered for approximately 5-12 minutes. (See package directions. Cooking time varies by size and shape.) 2 oz dry makes 1 cup cooked.

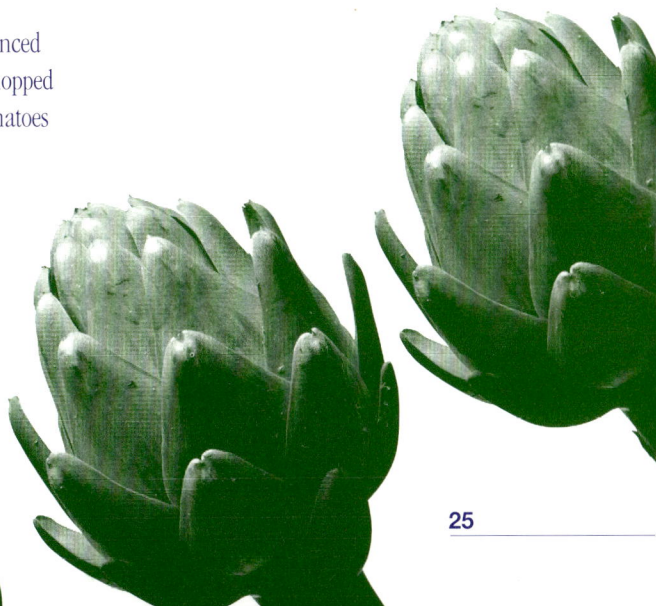

Nutritional Analyses

The recipes were analyzed using the Nutritionist IV Food Labeling program. Because precise nutrition information is not yet available on all foods, the numbers are approximate. Rather than "eating by number", the best way to eat a healthy diet is to enjoy the wide variety of foods that are naturally low in fat and high in nutrients and flavor. All of the recipes take this approach. Plant foods are emphasized and animal proteins are used in smaller amounts or are optional.

The nutritional analysis is based on five servings. Optional ingredients are not included. If more than one ingredient is suggested, the first one is used in the analysis. Reduced-sodium soy sauce and broth and reduced-fat cheeses and tofu were used for the nutritional analysis. Added salt was not included in the analysis. (One teaspoon has 2300 mg. of sodium).

Pasta

Asian
Serving Size: 1½ cups

Amount per serving
Calories 375   Calories from fat 45

	% Daily Value*
Total Fat 5g	8%
Saturated Fat 1g	5%
Cholesterol 25mg	8%
Sodium 420mg	18%
Total Carbohydrate 60g	20%
Dietary Fiber 3g	12%
Sugars 8g	
Protein 21g	

Vitamin A 120%   Vitamin C 40%
Calcium 6%   Iron 30%

Food Exchanges
2 vegetable, 3 bread, 1 meat, 1 fat

French
Serving Size: 1½ cups

Amount per serving
Calories 420   Calories from fat 20

	% Daily Value*
Total Fat 2g	3%
Saturated Fat .5g	2%
Cholesterol 25mg	8%
Sodium 370mg	15%
Total Carbohydrate 66g	22%
Dietary Fiber 2g	8%
Sugars 7g	
Protein 27g	

Vitamin A 15%   Vitamin C 35%
Calcium 25%   Iron 35%

Food Exchanges
3 vegetable, 3½ bread, 1 meat

Italian
Serving Size: 1½ cups

Amount per serving
Calories 400   Calories from fat 35

	% Daily Value*
Total Fat 4g	6%
Saturated Fat .5g	2%
Cholesterol 0mg	0%
Sodium 125mg	15%
Total Carbohydrate 68g	23%
Dietary Fiber 5g	20%
Sugars 9g	
Protein 17g	

Vitamin A 15%   Vitamin C 60%
Calcium 8%   Iron 35%

Food Exchanges
2 vegetable, 4 bread, 1 fat

Mexican
Serving Size: 1½ cups

Amount per serving
Calories 350   Calories from fat 20

	% Daily Value*
Total Fat 2g	3%
Saturated Fat .5g	2%
Cholesterol 0mg	0%
Sodium 400mg	16%
Total Carbohydrate 67g	22%
Dietary Fiber 6g	24%
Sugars 8g	
Protein 15g	

Vitamin A 15%   Vitamin C 170%
Calcium 8%   Iron 40%

Food Exchanges
2 vegetable, 4 bread

Spanish
Serving Size: 1½ cups

Amount per serving
Calories 380   Calories from fat 35

	% Daily Value*
Total Fat 4g	6%
Saturated Fat .5g	2%
Cholesterol 15mg	5%
Sodium 65mg	3%
Total Carbohydrate 64g	21%
Dietary Fiber 4g	16%
Sugars 7g	
Protein 21g	

Vitamin A 8%   Vitamin C 260%
Calcium 6%   Iron 25%

Food Exchanges
3 vegetable, 3½ bread, 1 meat

Pizza

Asian
Serving Size: ⅕ pizza

Amount per serving
Calories 330   Calories from fat 25

	% Daily Value*
Total Fat 3g	5%
Saturated Fat .5g	2%
Cholesterol 0mg	0%
Sodium 590mg	25%
Total Carbohydrate 65g	22%
Dietary Fiber 3g	12%
Sugars 8g	
Protein 14g	

Vitamin A 8%   Vitamin C 100%
Calcium 10%   Iron 30%

Food Exchanges
2 vegetable, 3 bread, 1 fat

Greek
Serving Size: ⅕ pizza

Amount per serving
Calories 330   Calories from fat 40

	% Daily Value*
Total Fat 5g	8%
Saturated Fat .5g	2%
Cholesterol 0mg	0%
Sodium 320mg	13%
Total Carbohydrate 63g	21%
Dietary Fiber 2g	8%
Sugars 15g	
Protein 10g	

Vitamin A 15%   Vitamin C 70%
Calcium 8%   Iron 20%

Food Exchanges
1 fruit, 3 bread, 1 fat

Italian
Serving Size: ⅕ pizza

Amount per serving
Calories 360   Calories from fat 40

	% Daily Value*
Total Fat 4g	6%
Saturated Fat .5g	2%
Cholesterol 10mg	3%
Sodium 800mg	30%
Total Carbohydrate 66g	22%
Dietary Fiber 4g	16%
Sugars 6g	
Protein 19g	

Vitamin A 130%   Vitamin C 30%
Calcium 8%   Iron 25%

Food Exchanges
3 vegetable, 3 bread, 1 fat

Mediterranean
Serving Size: ⅕ pizza

Amount per serving
Calories 320   Calories from fat 60

	% Daily Value*
Total Fat 6g	9%
Saturated Fat 1.5g	8%
Cholesterol 5mg	2%
Sodium 500mg	21%
Total Carbohydrate 55g	18%
Dietary Fiber 2g	8%
Sugars 6g	
Protein 13g	

Vitamin A 8%   Vitamin C 25%
Calcium 15%   Iron 20%

Food Exchanges
1 vegetable, 3 bread, 1 fat

Mexican
Serving Size: ⅕ pizza

Amount per serving
Calories 270   Calories from fat 60

	% Daily Value*
Total Fat 7g	11%
Saturated Fat 2.5g	12%
Cholesterol 15mg	5%
Sodium 800mg	30%
Total Carbohydrate 41g	14%
Dietary Fiber 5g	20%
Sugars 3g	
Protein 13g	

Vitamin A 15%   Vitamin C 150%
Calcium 25%   Iron 20%

Food Exchanges
1 vegetable, 2 bread, 1 meat, 1 fat

Sauté

Asian
Serving Size: 1½ cups

Amount per serving

Calories 320 Calories from fat 40

	% Daily Value*
Total Fat 4g	**6**%
Saturated Fat .5g	**2**%
Cholesterol 10mg	**3**%
Sodium 320mg	**13**%
Total Carbohydrate 58g	**19**%
Dietary Fiber 5g	**20**%
Sugars 9g	
Protein 14g	

Vitamin A 240%   Vitamin C 80%
Calcium 8%   Iron 15%

Food Exchanges
2 vegetable, 3 bread, 1 meat

Indian
Serving Size: 1½ cups

Amount per serving

Calories 330 Calories from fat 60

	% Daily Value*
Total Fat 7g	**11**%
Saturated Fat .5g	**2**%
Sodium 110mg	**5**%
Total Carbohydrate 64g	**21**%
Dietary Fiber 5g	**20**%
Sugars 13g	
Protein 7g	

Vitamin A 240%   Vitamin C 25%
Calcium 8%   Iron 10%

Food Exchanges
1 vegetable, 1 fruit, 3 bread, 1 fat

Indonesian
Serving Size: 1½ cups

Amount per serving

Calories 330 Calories from fat 45

	% Daily Value*
Total Fat 5g	**8**%
Saturated Fat 1g	**5**%
Sodium 270mg	**11**%
Total Carbohydrate 66g	**22**%
Dietary Fiber 5g	**20**%
Sugars 12g	
Protein 9g	

Vitamin A 25%   Vitamin C 70%
Calcium 10%   Iron 20%

Food Exchanges
2 vegetable, 3 bread, 1 fat

Mexican
Serving Size: 1½ cups

Amount per serving

Calories 340 Calories from fat 60

	% Daily Value*
Total Fat 6g	**9**%
Saturated Fat .5g	**2**%
Sodium 300mg	**12**%
Total Carbohydrate 64g	**21**%
Dietary Fiber 7g	**28**%
Sugars 6g	
Protein 10g	

Vitamin A 8%   Vitamin C 220%
Calcium 8%   Iron 20%

Food Exchanges
3 vegetable, 3 bread, 1 fat

Moroccan
Serving Size: 1½ cups

Amount per serving

Calories 310 Calories from fat 20

	% Daily Value*
Total Fat 2g	**3**%
Saturated Fat .5g	**2**%
Cholesterol 25mg	**8**%
Sodium 200mg	**8**%
Total Carbohydrate 53g	**18**%
Dietary Fiber 11g	**44**%
Sugars 6g	
Protein 18g	

Vitamin A 8%   Vitamin C 130%
Calcium 8%   Iron 10%

Food Exchanges
2 vegetable, 3 bread, 1 meat

Stir Fry

Indian
Serving Size: 1½ cups

Amount per serving

Calories 320 Calories from fat 60

	% Daily Value*
Total Fat 7g	**11**%
Saturated Fat .5g	**2**%
Cholesterol 0mg	**0**%
Sodium 20mg	**1**%
Total Carbohydrate 55g	**18**%
Dietary Fiber 2g	**8**%
Sugars 5g	
Protein 8g	

Vitamin A 20%   Vitamin C 160%
Calcium 15%   Iron 20%

Food Exchanges
1 vegetable, 3 bread, 1 fat

Italian
Serving Size: 2 cups

Amount per serving

Calories 380 Calories from fat 60

	% Daily Value*
Total Fat 6g	**9**%
Saturated Fat 1g	**10**%
Cholesterol 5mg	**2**%
Sodium 210mg	**9**%
Total Carbohydrate 65g	**22**%
Dietary Fiber 5g	**20**%
Sugars 5g	
Protein 15g	

Vitamin A 25%   Vitamin C 80%
Calcium 15%   Iron 25%

Food Exchanges
1 vegetable, 4 bread, 1 fat

Japanese
Serving Size: 2 cups

Amount per serving

Calories 360 Calories from fat 50

	% Daily Value*
Total Fat 6g	**9**%
Saturated Fat 1g	**5**%
Cholesterol 0mg	**0**%
Sodium 150mg	**6**%
Total Carbohydrate 64g	**21**%
Dietary Fiber 5g	**20**%
Sugars 5g	
Protein 13g	

Vitamin A 15%   Vitamin C 140%
Calcium 8%   Iron 25%

Food Exchanges
1 vegetable, 4 bread, 1 fat

Mexican
Serving Size: 1½ cups

Amount per serving

Calories 320 Calories from fat 60

	% Daily Value*
Total Fat 7g	**11**%
Saturated Fat .5g	**2**%
Cholesterol 0mg	**0**%
Sodium 460mg	**19**%
Total Carbohydrate 57g	**19**%
Dietary Fiber 7g	**28**%
Sugars 4g	
Protein 9g	

Vitamin A 120%   Vitamin C 60%
Calcium 8%   Iron 15%

Food Exchanges
2 vegetable, 3 bread, 1 fat

Thai
Serving Size: 1½ cups

Amount per serving

Calories 320 Calories from fat 50

	% Daily Value*
Total Fat 5g	**8**%
Saturated Fat 1g	**5**%
Cholesterol 0mg	**0**%
Sodium 680mg	**28**%
Total Carbohydrate 61g	**20**%
Dietary Fiber 5g	**20**%
Sugars 7g	
Protein 7g	

Vitamin A 120%   Vitamin C 90%
Calcium 15%   Iron 20%

Food Exchanges
2 vegetable, 3 bread, 1 fat

Oven Baked Dishes

French
Serving Size: 1/5 recipe

Amount per serving

Calories 230 Calories from fat 45

	% Daily Value*
Total Fat 5g	**8**%
Saturated Fat 3g	**15**%
Cholesterol 10mg	**3**%
Sodium 300mg	**12**%
Total Carbohydrate 34g	**11**%
Dietary Fiber 5g	**20**%
Sugars 8g	
Protein 11g	

Vitamin A 15%   Vitamin C 90%
Calcium 30%   Iron 10%

Food Exchanges
2 vegetable, 1½ bread, 1 fat

Indian
Serving Size: 1/5 recipe

Amount per serving

Calories 460 Calories from fat 70

	% Daily Value*
Total Fat 8g	**12**%
Saturated Fat 2g	**10**%
Cholesterol 10mg	**0**%
Sodium 65mg	**3**%
Total Carbohydrate 86g	**29**%
Dietary Fiber 10g	**40**%
Sugars 13g	
Protein 13g	

Vitamin A 350%   Vitamin C 60%
Calcium 8%   Iron 25%

Food Exchanges
4 vegetable, 4 bread, 1 fat

Italian
Serving Size: 1/5 recipe

Amount per serving

Calories 260 Calories from fat 45

	% Daily Value*
Total Fat 5g	**8**%
Saturated Fat .5g	**2**%
Cholesterol 10mg	**3**%
Sodium 180mg	**8**%
Total Carbohydrate 42g	**14**%
Dietary Fiber 5g	**20**%
Sugars 3g	
Protein 13g	

Vitamin A 30%   Vitamin C 80%
Calcium 20%   Iron 25%

Food Exchanges
3 vegetable, 1 bread, 1 meat, 1 fat

Mediterranean
Serving Size: 1/5 recipe

Amount per serving

Calories 280 Calories from fat 90

	% Daily Value*
Total Fat 9g	**13**%
Saturated Fat 4.5g	**22**%
Cholesterol 25mg	**8**%
Sodium 710mg	**30**%
Total Carbohydrate 41g	**14**%
Dietary Fiber 7g	**28**%
Sugars 4g	
Protein 12g	

Vitamin A 70%   Vitamin C 60%
Calcium 30%   Iron 20%

Food Exchanges
2 vegetable, 2 bread, 2 fat

Mexican
Serving Size: 1/5 recipe

Amount per serving

Calories 280 Calories from fat C0

	% Daily Value*
Total Fat 7g	**11**%
Saturated Fat 1.5g	**8**%
Cholesterol 10mg	**3**%
Sodium 600mg	**25**%
Total Carbohydrate 39g	**13**%
Dietary Fiber 7g	**28**%
Sugars 3g	
Protein 12g	

Vitamin A 15%   Vitamin C 170%
Calcium 30%   Iron 10%

Food Exchanges
1 vegetable, 2 bread, 1 meat, 1 fat

Soup

California Vegetable
Serving Size: 1½ cups
Amount per serving
Calories 100 Calories from fat 25
% Daily Value*
Total Fat 3g	5%
Saturated Fat 1.5g	8%
Sodium 320mg	13%
Total Carbohydrate 16g	5%
Dietary Fiber 2g	8%
Sugars 5g	
Protein 2g	

Vitamin A 60%   Vitamin C 20%
Calcium 4%   Iron 8%

Food Exchanges
1½ vegetable, ½ bread

Indian Curried Lentil
Serving Size: 1½ cups
Amount per serving
Calories 140 Calories from fat 25
% Daily Value*
Total Fat 2g	3%
Saturated Fat 1.5g	8%
Sodium 105mg	4%
Total Carbohydrate 19g	6%
Dietary Fiber 2g	8%
Sugars 3g	
Protein 8g	

Vitamin A 10%   Vitamin C 4%
Calcium 6%   Iron 15%

Food Exchanges
½ vegetable, 1 bread

Mediterranean Onion
Serving Size: 1½ cups
Amount per serving
Calories 130 Calories from fat 45
% Daily Value*
Total Fat 4g	6%
Saturated Fat 1g	5%
Sodium 190mg	8%
Total Carbohydrate 16g	5%
Dietary Fiber 2g	8%
Sugars 6g	
Protein 6g	

Vitamin A 4%   Vitamin C 20%
Calcium 10%   Iron 8%

Food Exchanges
2 vegetable, ½ bread, ½ fat

Middle Eastern Hummus
Serving Size: 1½ cups
Amount per serving
Calories 130 Calories from fat 45
% Daily Value*
Total Fat 4g	6%
Saturated Fat 1.5g	8%
Sodium 320mg	13%
Total Carbohydrate 15g	5%
Dietary Fiber 3g	12%
Sugars 2g	
Protein 6g	

Vitamin A 20%   Vitamin C 15%
Calcium 4%   Iron 15%

Food Exchanges
½ vegetable, 1 bread, ½ fat

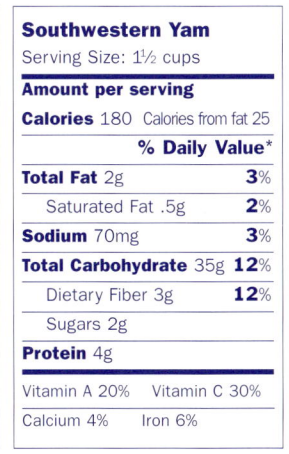

Southwestern Yam
Serving Size: 1½ cups
Amount per serving
Calories 180 Calories from fat 25
% Daily Value*
Total Fat 2g	3%
Saturated Fat .5g	2%
Sodium 70mg	3%
Total Carbohydrate 35g	12%
Dietary Fiber 3g	12%
Sugars 2g	
Protein 4g	

Vitamin A 20%   Vitamin C 30%
Calcium 4%   Iron 6%

Food Exchanges
½ vegetable, 2 bread

Grain

Asian Rice
Serving Size: 1 cup
Amount per serving
Calories 240 Calories from fat 35
% Daily Value*
Total Fat 4g	6%
Saturated Fat 1g	5%
Sodium 110mg	5%
Total Carbohydrate 45g	15%
Dietary Fiber 1g	4%
Sugars 2g	
Protein 4g	

Vitamin A 40%   Vitamin C 4%
Calcium 4%   Iron 15%

Food Exchanges
½ vegetable, 2½ bread, ½ fat

Italian Rice
Serving Size: 1 cup
Amount per serving
Calories 240 Calories from fat 45
% Daily Value*
Total Fat 4g	6%
Saturated Fat 1g	5%
Sodium 65mg	3%
Total Carbohydrate 44g	15%
Dietary Fiber 1g	4%
Sugars 1g	
Protein 5g	

Vitamin A 0%   Vitamin C 20%
Calcium 4%   Iron 10%

Food Exchanges
2½ bread, 1 fat

Mexican Rice
Serving Size: 1¼ cup
Amount per serving
Calories 260 Calories from fat 25
% Daily Value*
Total Fat 3g	5%
Saturated Fat 1g	5%
Sodium 25mg	1%
Total Carbohydrate 51g	17%
Dietary Fiber 3g	12%
Sugars 2g	
Protein 7g	

Vitamin A 8%   Vitamin C 4%
Calcium 4%   Iron 15%

Food Exchanges
½ vegetable, 3 bread, ½ fat

Moroccan Couscous
Serving Size: 1 cup
Amount per serving
Calories 240 Calories from fat 45
% Daily Value*
Total Fat 4g	6%
Saturated Fat .5g	2%
Sodium 70mg	3%
Total Carbohydrate 42g	14%
Dietary Fiber 8g	32%
Sugars 5g	
Protein 7g	

Vitamin A 0%   Vitamin C 15%
Calcium 4%   Iron 8%

Food Exchanges
½ vegetable, 2½ bread, 1 fat

Southwestern Quinoa
Serving Size: 1 cup
Amount per serving
Calories 230 Calories from fat 70
% Daily Value*
Total Fat 7g	10%
Saturated Fat 1g	5%
Sodium 30mg	1%
Total Carbohydrate 34g	11%
Dietary Fiber 3g	12%
Sugars 2g	
Protein 7g	

Vitamin A 8%   Vitamin C 4%
Calcium 4%   Iron 25%

Food Exchanges
½ vegetable, 2 bread, 1½ fat

Veggies

Asian Carrots
Serving Size: 1 cup
Amount per serving
Calories 80 Calories from fat 25
% Daily Value*
Total Fat 2g	3%
Saturated Fat 1g	5%
Sodium 55mg	2%
Total Carbohydrate 10g	3%
Dietary Fiber 5g	20%
Sugars 7g	
Protein 1g	

Vitamin A 200%   Vitamin C 15%
Calcium 2%   Iron 6%

Food Exchanges
2 vegetable, ½ fat

Mediterranean Broccoli
Serving Size: ¾ cup
Amount per serving
Calories 60 Calories from fat 25
% Daily Value*
Total Fat 3g	5%
Saturated Fat 1g	5%
Sodium 15mg	1%
Total Carbohydrate 4g	1%
Dietary Fiber 2g	8%
Protein 6g	

Vitamin A 8%   Vitamin C 170%
Calcium 8%   Iron 8%

Food Exchanges
1 vegetable, ½ fat

Italian Zucchini
Serving Size: 1 cup
Amount per serving
Calories 50 Calories from fat 20
% Daily Value*
Total Fat 2.5g	4%
Saturated Fat 1g	5%
Sodium 10mg	0%
Total Carbohydrate 8g	3%
Dietary Fiber 2g	8%
Sugars 4g	
Protein 1g	

Vitamin A 30%   Vitamin C 15%
Calcium 4%   Iron 4%

Food Exchanges
1½ vegetable, ½ fat

Mexican Peppers & Onions
Serving Size: 1 cup
Amount per serving
Calories 60 Calories from fat 25
% Daily Value*
Total Fat 1g	5%
Saturated Fat 1g	5%
Sodium 0mg	0%
Total Carbohydrate 7g	2%
Dietary Fiber 3g	12%
Sugars 5g	
Protein 2g	

Vitamin A 4%   Vitamin C 180%
Calcium 2%   Iron 4%

Food Exchanges
1½ vegetable, ½ fat

Irish Green Beans
Serving Size: 1 cup
Amount per serving
Calories 60 Calories from fat 0
% Daily Value*
Total Fat 0g	0%
Saturated Fat 0g	0%
Sodium 10mg	0%
Total Carbohydrate 13g	4%
Dietary Fiber 3g	12%
Protein 2g	

Vitamin A 8%   Vitamin C 25%
Calcium 6%   Iron 10%

Food Exchanges
2 vegetables

Chicken/Fish/Soy

Asian Tofu
Serving Size: 3.2 oz

Amount per serving

Calories 110 Calories from fat 50

% Daily Value*

Total Fat 6g	**9%**
Saturated Fat 1g	**5%**
Sodium 220mg	**9%**
Total Carbohydrate 4g	**1%**
Dietary Fiber 2g	**8%**
Protein 9g	

Vitamin A 0%   Vitamin C 0%
Calcium 4%   Iron 8%

Food Exchanges
2 meat, 1 fat

Cajun Chicken
Serving Size: 3 oz

Amount per serving

Calories 130 Calories from fat 50

% Daily Value*

Total Fat 5g	**8%**
Saturated Fat 1.5g	**8%**
Cholesterol 70mg	**23%**
Sodium 240mg	**10%**
Total Carbohydrate 2g	**1%**
Protein 16g	

Vitamin A 2%   Vitamin C 4%
Calcium 0%   Iron 4%

Food Exchanges
3 meat

Cuban Fish
Serving Size: 3 oz

Amount per serving

Calories 90 Calories from fat 15

% Daily Value*

Total Fat 1.5g	**2%**
Saturated Fat 1g	**5%**
Sodium 90mg	**4%**
Total Carbohydrate 2g	**1%**
Protein 18g	

Vitamin A 2%   Vitamin C 6%
Calcium 4%   Iron 2%

Food Exchanges
3 meat

French Salmon
Serving Size: 3 oz

Amount per serving

Calories 120 Calories from fat 35

% Daily Value*

Total Fat 4g	**6%**
Saturated Fat 1.5g	**8%**
Cholesterol 55mg	**18%**
Sodium 70mg	**3%**
Total Carbohydrate 0g	**0%**
Protein 21g	

Vitamin A 4%   Vitamin C 0%
Calcium 0%   Iron 4%

Food Exchanges
3 meat

Mediterranean Chicken
Serving Size: 3 oz

Amount per serving

Calories 140 Calories from fat 60

% Daily Value*

Total Fat 5g	**8%**
Saturated Fat 1.5g	**8%**
Cholesterol 70mg	**23%**
Sodium 55mg	**2%**
Total Carbohydrate 3g	**1%**
Protein 16g	

Vitamin A 0%   Vitamin C 4%
Calcium 0%   Iron 4%

Food Exchanges
3 meat

Dessert

Hawaiian Medley
Serving Size: 1 cup

Amount per serving

Calories 120 Calories from fat 20

% Daily Value*

Total Fat 1g	**1%**
Saturated Fat 0g	**0%**
Sodium 0mg	**0%**
Total Carbohydrate 27g	**9%**
Dietary Fiber 1g	**4%**
Sugars 7g	
Protein 2g	

Vitamin A 4%   Vitamin C 15%
Calcium 2%   Iron 4%

Food Exchanges
2 fruit

Italian Bella Frutta
Serving Size: 1 cup

Amount per serving

Calories 80 Calories from fat 10

% Daily Value*

Total Fat 1g	**2%**
Saturated Fat 0g	**0%**
Sodium 0mg	**0%**
Total Carbohydrate 17g	**6%**
Dietary Fiber 3g	**12%**
Sugars 2g	
Protein 1g	

Vitamin A 0%   Vitamin C 15%
Calcium 0%   Iron 4%

Food Exchanges
1 fruit

French Citrus Supreme
Serving Size: 1 cup

Amount per serving

Calories 70 Calories from fat 10

% Daily Value*

Total Fat 1g	**2%**
Saturated Fat .5g	**2%**
Sodium 0mg	**0%**
Total Carbohydrate 14g	**5%**
Dietary Fiber 10g	**40%**
Sugars 13g	
Protein 2g	

Vitamin A 0%   Vitamin C 130%
Calcium 6%   Iron 4%

Food Exchanges
1 fruit

American Apple Berry
Serving Size: 1 cup

Amount per serving

Calories 130 Calories from fat 15

% Daily Value*

Total Fat 1.5g	**2%**
Saturated Fat .5g	**2%**
Sodium 15mg	**1%**
Total Carbohydrate 28g	**9%**
Dietary Fiber 4g	**16%**
Sugars 14g	
Protein 1g	

Vitamin A 2%   Vitamin C 80%
Calcium 4%   Iron 4%

Food Exchanges
2 fruit

New Zealand Delight
Serving Size: 1 cup

Amount per serving

Calories 110 Calories from fat 20

% Daily Value*

Total Fat 1g	**1%**
Saturated Fat 1g	**5%**
Sodium 5mg	**0%**
Total Carbohydrate 20g	**7%**
Dietary Fiber 5g	**20%**
Sugars 11g	
Protein 3g	

Vitamin A 0%   Vitamin C 170%
Calcium 8%   Iron 6%

Food Exchanges
1¼ fruit

Food & Nutrition Resources

Associations

American Dietetic Association
216 W. Jackson Blvd., Suite 800
Chicago, IL 60606-6995
1-800-366-1635
www.eatright.org (has links to other health and nutrition websites)

5 A Day
www.5aday.com

Newsletters

Environmental Nutrition
P.O. Box 420451
Palm Coast, FL 32142-0451
800-829-5384

Nutrition Action Health Letter
Center for Science in the Public Interest
1875 Connecticut Ave., N.W., Suite 300
Washington, D.C. 20009-5728
www.cspinet.org (has links to other health and nutrition websites)

Tufts University Health & Nutrition Letter
P.O. Box 57857
Boulder, CO 80322-7857
1-800-274-7581
www.healthletter.tufts.edu (has links to other health and nutrition websites)

University of California, Berkeley Wellness Letter
P.O. Box 420148
Palm Coast, FL 32142
800-829-9170

To order additional copies of Quickflip to Delicious Dinners, please send the coupon below to: Nutrition Connections, P.O. Box 21175, Boulder, CO 80308. (Call 888-554-3547 for quantity and wholesale price list.)

- -

Please send:

_____ copies of Quickflip to Delicious Dinners @ $17.95 each $ _____

3% sales tax (Colorado residents only) $ _____

Shipping $2.95 for first book, .75 each additional book $ _____

TOTAL $ _____

Send to:

Name _____

Address _____

City/State/Zip _____

Telephone _____

Payment:

☐ Check or Money Order enclosed (payable to Nutrition Connections)

☐ Visa   ☐ MasterCard

Card Number: _____ Exp. date ___/___

Name on card: _____

Signature: _____